One Plus One
Equals
Emotional Survival

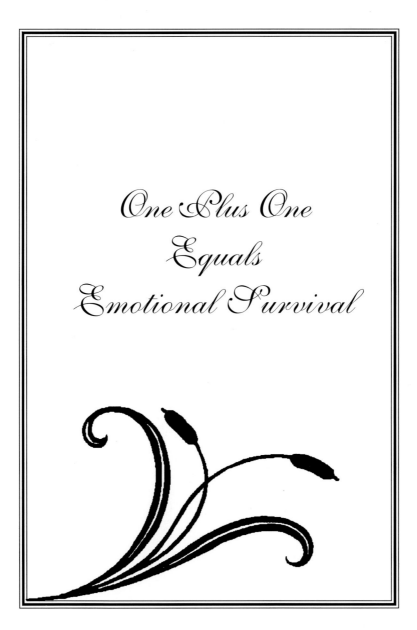

Helping Your Mate Face Breast Cancer

Tips for becoming an effective support partner for the one you love during the breast cancer experience

Judy C. Kneece, RN, OCN
Breast Health Specialist

Edu&Care Publishing®
P. O. Box 280305
Columbia, S. C. 29228

4th Revised Edition 2001; 3rd Revised Edition 1999; 2nd Edition 1997; 1st Edition 1995.
ISBN 1-886665-11-7
Library of Congress Card Number: 98-93958
Printed in the United States of America
Published by EduCare Publishing
To order:
    EduCare Publishing
    P. O. Box 280305
    Columbia, S. C. 29228
    Voice: 803-796-6100 or Fax: 803-796-4150
    Internet: http://www.cancerhelp.com/
    E-Mail: educare@ix.netcom.com

Publisher's Cataloging-in-Publication

Kneece, Judy C.
    Helping your mate face breast cancer : tips for
becoming an effective support partner for the one you love
during the breast cancer experience / Judy C. Kneece. --
4th rev. ed.
    p. cm.
    Includes bibliographical references and index.
    ISBN: 1-886665-11-7
    Preassigned LCCN: 99-93958

    1. Breast--Cancer--Patients. 2. Cancer--Patients--Family
relationships. I. Title.

    RC280.B8K64 2001   616.99'449
                             QBI01-121

Dedication

This book is dedicated to all the patients and their mates who have shared openly and honestly about their physical and emotional journeys with breast cancer. Their courage serves as a source of inspiration and proof that facing a crisis together can make a relationship even more meaningful and fulfilling.

A special debt of gratitude is extended to Cindy Dreher, MPH, MAT, for her visionary efforts in women's health issues by recognizing the acute need for the psychosocial support of patients and their families during the breast cancer experience. It was through her experience as a support partner for her mother, Nell Dreher, and her best friend, Francee Lang Giles, that Cindy personally experienced the great need of families and friends for education and support. It is also through her personal support that I had the opportunity to develop a psychosocial program to meet this need. Her influence is evident throughout this book and my work with breast cancer patients.

To Tom Winnett, I owe my motivation to begin programs for the support partner. After speaking to a large group of women, Tom looked at me with tears in his eyes and said, "Women have many places to go for help, but where is a man supposed to get help? . . . We hurt too." Thanks, Tom, for being frank and a catalyst for including the support partner and family in all of my work.

In addition, I dedicate this book to Bill, my support partner, whose words of encouragement and support have made my work with breast cancer patients, their support partners and this book possible.

Acknowledgments

A special word of appreciation to the following people for their contributions to this work:

Cindy Dreher, MPH, MAT, for her support, encouragement and valuable input concerning the psychosocial issues of the breast cancer experience.

Tom Rice, Ph.D., University of South Carolina professor, and **Diane Rice**, breast cancer survivor, for sharing openly and reviewing the manuscript.

Reverend Sinclair Lewis, M.Div., D.D., Methodist pastor, and **Betty Lewis**, breast cancer survivor, for their manuscript review.

Dr. Marianna Maldonado, Psychiatrist and breast cancer survivor, for her insightful expertise in the psychological recovery from breast cancer and her review of the manuscript.

Dr. Henry Leis, Breast Surgeon, for his encouragement and surgical input.

Dr. Frederick Greene, Breast Surgeon, for his surgical input.

Dr. Rosemary Lambert-Falls, Medical Oncologist, for her oncology review and encouragement.

Dr. Elizabeth Wofford, Pathologist, for reviewing the pathology section.

Dr. Ervin Shaw, Pathologist, for reviewing the pathology section.

Jerry Kennedy, MN, RNCS, for her nursing input and encouragement to me in my work with cancer patients.

Al Barrineau, support partner, for his commentary on his experience during his mate's breast cancer experience.

Tricia Carter Brown, Editor, and for her encouragement.

Tom Smith, Ph. D., and **Carolyn B. Brennan,** Editorial Consultants

Debra Strange, Art Illustrations

Contents

═══════════

Support Partners
provide an inexpressible
comfort of feeling totally
safe with
another person.

About The Author

Judy Kneece, RN, OCN, is a certified oncology nurse with a specialty in breast cancer and a
MammaCare® Specialist. She presently serves as
an international Breast Health Consultant for hospitals and breast health centers in the educational
and psychosocial needs of breast cancer patients
and their families. She implements a program of
comprehensive education, training nurses to fill the
breast health education role, and sets up a com-
plete program of support for the entire family.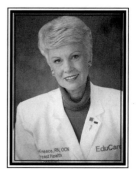

Her background as a Breast Health Specialist working in a hospital served as a catalyst for her insights into the needs of women and
their families during the breast cancer experience. Judy has personally intervened at the time of diagnosis with hundreds of patients and
their families, providing emotional support and education about the
disease, treatments and recovery. She developed and led support
groups for patients and their mates and followed the patients throughout the recovery experience.

She is also the author of *Your Breast Cancer Treatment Handbook*, a book for breast cancer patients, *Finding A Lump In Your
Breast—Where To Go . . . What To Do*, *Solving the Mystery of Breast
Pain*, *Solving the Mystery of Breast Discharge* and of a computer
program featuring over 240 patient teaching sheets on breast health for
clinics, hospitals and physician's offices. She presently serves as Managed Care Breast Health Editor for *Administrative Radiology Journal*
and Managing Editor for the *Breast Center Bulletin*. Judy serves on the
Board of Directors and as secretary for the National Consortium of Breast
Centers. She speaks widely on the topic of breast cancer education
and triumphant survivorship.

"Breast cancer does not happen in a social vacuum. It happens in
a family. Breast cancer is a family illness. Everyone in the family
suffers, and support tools for recovery are essential for all members
to successfully master the crisis. With proper education and support
the family unit can emerge emotionally intact," shares Judy.

Let me introduce:

Al Barrineau, support partner

When I finished this manuscript, it was not really complete. It lacked the voice of a peer. You, a new support partner, needed to hear from one who had personally experienced the feelings, fears and joys of the support role.

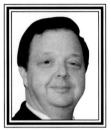

I had the privilege of working with Al and his wife, Harriett, for three years as they worked through the breast cancer experience. Involved with them in their journey were four sons, ages 14 to 21. Breast cancer is a family affair. The entire family feels the effects.

Harriett was diagnosed with a breast cancer which required a mastectomy. Eventually, she underwent a second mastectomy and bilateral reconstruction. During this time they were active in support groups, sharing their pain during their journey and offering encouragement to others.

I asked Al to serve as the voice of a peer, drawing from his diary of innermost thoughts, fears and reactions during this time. Sprinkled throughout this book are his feelings, sharing intimate experiences to help you. Hopefully, showing how one couple successfully maneuvered through the breast cancer experience will give you the courage to know that you and the one you love can also make it.

Helping the one you love face breast cancer is a challenge. It is a challenge that requires a commitment of support, and support has been proven as one of the most important components for a successful recovery. Therefore, you have inherited a very important role– support partner.

Introduction

=======

*" 'I'm sorry; the tumor is malignant. Your wife has
breast cancer.' Those few words sent a chill through
me. Those words would test all human emotion in
me during the weeks and months to come."*
~Al Barrineau, support partner

Cancer. The most terrifying word in the English language. When
you hear it applied to someone you love, its meaning amplifies and
grows to paralyzing proportions. Shock, fear, confusion, and denial
absorb your mind and body. There is no "Cancer 101" training to
prepare you to know what to do or say, where to go for help, or how
to be the most support to the one you love. You have inherited a new
role–support partner. It is a role with many new demands.

A breast cancer diagnosis stresses and shakes the equilibrium of a
relationship. Dr. Marilyn T. Oberst sums up the stress placed on those
who inherit a support role. "Learning to live with cancer is clearly
no easy task," she says. "Learning to live with someone else's cancer
may be even more **difficult**, precisely because no one recognizes
just how **hard** it really is to **deal** with **someone else's cancer**." Living with someone else's cancer is a challenge; but it is a challenge
which can be mastered successfully. The key is to learn how to manage the emotional and physical demands.

Many examples quoted in this book are from the most common
support partner, a spouse. However, the same principles of support
apply to any relationship that serves as the primary support person
for a breast cancer patient. Often this may be a parent, sibling, or a
friend serving in the role of primary support.

This book was written from my experience working with and observing hundreds of breast cancer patients and their support partners as they worked through the cancer experience. My work allowed me to maintain an ongoing relationship with the patient and her partner throughout the course of her treatment and recovery. My goal is to help you understand the challenge of living with the pain of someone else's breast cancer diagnosis and to assist you in becoming a more effective support person.

Many patients and their support partners have openly shared with me their pain and efforts to make "sense out of a senseless situation" in hopes that the breast cancer experience will be more positive for those like you who inherit the role. It has been said, "If you want to find your way out of a forest, it is not as helpful to ask a forester, who knows all about the trees, but to ask someone who was lost but managed to find the way out of the forest." This book is from those who managed to find their own way through the forest of the breast cancer experience.

This book is not designed as a comprehensive manual on coping. Instead, it is a revelation of life experiences from patients, their support partners and my clinical experience. I urge you to reach out to other professionals, counselors, physicians, nurses and support groups to complete your understanding of the "support" role.

Through this book you will also gain an understanding of the basics of the breast cancer treatment process. You will learn effective and supportive techniques to ease the process and find additional resources available to assist you and your family. The support role is not an easy one; but, it is one from which you can learn and grow as you provide one of the most powerful tools for your mate's recovery from breast cancer—effective support.

My best wishes for a rewarding support experience,

Judy Kneece

Support Partners
assist you with their hands and
hearts in times of adversity.

*"We gain perspective by
having someone at our side.
We gain objectivity.
We gain courage in threatening
situations. Having others near
tempers our dogmatism and
softens our intolerance.
We gain another opinion.
We gain what today
is called input."*

~ Chuck Swindoll

Chapter 1

What Is a
Support Partner?

*"My wife has always been the caretaker and care giver
in our family. She nursed us during illness, praised
our accomplishments, encouraged us in our trials, paid
the compliments, initiated the hugging–now the roles
were reversed. She needed these things from me. My
world had been shaken to the core. I wasn't sure I
could be what she needed."*

~Al Barrineau, support partner

You have inherited a new role, support partner for a breast cancer patient. What does the role of support partner mean? The role is best described by the *American Heritage Dictionary* (Third Edition).

sup·port v. 1. To bear the weight of, especially from below. 2. To hold in position so as to keep from falling, sinking, or slipping. 3. To be capable of bearing; withstand. 4. To keep from weakening or failing; strengthen. 5. To provide for or maintain, by supplying with money or necessities. 6. To furnish corroborating evidence for. 7. To aid the cause, policy, or interests of. 8. To endure; tolerate. 9. To act in a secondary or subordinate role to (a leading performer).

sup·port n. 1. a. The act of supporting. b. The state of being supported. 2. One that supports. 3. Maintenance, as of a family, with the necessities of life.

part·ner n. 1. One that is united or associated with another or others in an activity or a sphere of common interest. a. A spouse.

A support partner is a stabilizing force during a crisis, someone bound to another by a relationship or a common bond of interest. Support partners stand alongside the ones they love, sharing the emotional and physical burden as a stabilizing force. The role is a subordinate role, in that the patient takes the lead role in making decisions and sets the emotional tone. However, the support partner is the one who provides the fertile atmosphere of caring, who assists in information-gathering, fosters hope and assures the partner of their commitment for the duration of the crisis. The role of support partner is as important as any medical treatment the patient will receive. The gift of your support can make the difference in her physical and emotional recovery.

The following chapters include ways others have successfully filled this role. I challenge you to learn from those who have shared and to add your own inventive methods of support. I wish you a very rewarding support-role experience.

Remember

→ **Your role as a support partner is one of the most important components for the emotional recovery of the one you love.**

Chapter 2

The Initial Diagnosis

"Shock and fear best describe my first reaction. This was only supposed to happen to other women–not my wife. We were both in a daze. But one thing was for sure; my wife and I were in this together from the start."
~Al Barrineau, support partner

"You have breast cancer" are four words which forever change lives. The patient as well as those closest to her are suddenly faced with an unexpected challenge. Unplanned. Unprepared. Helpless. Confused. Yet, in the midst of all the emotions is the urgent need to make critical decisions about treatment.

The time from diagnosis through surgery is considered an acute phase of adjustment for the patient, partner and family members. During this time you and your partner will be required to learn about the disease, its treatments, emotions and effective communication skills. Your goal is to successfully maneuver through the experience and emerge emotionally intact. How this is accomplished will differ, based on the personality of the patient, your personality and both of your previous problem-solving and coping experiences. Even though relationship dynamics may differ, many problems and their solutions are common for the patient and for you, the support person.

During an unexpected crisis, there are some general physical and emotional changes which may occur in you or your mate. It is helpful to know that these symptoms are all signs of stress. Changes which you or your mate may experience:

- ◆ Body—headaches, feelings of exhaustion, stomach problems, minor pains, decreased resistance to colds, flu, etc.
- ◆ Mind—negative thoughts, confusion, difficulty concentrating, sleeplessness, forgetting details, mind going blank, lower productivity
- ◆ Feelings—anxiety, anger, fear, frustration, emotional withdrawal

Either you or your partner may experience these symptoms of stress in varying degrees. They are not a result of illness, but of a natural reaction during a crisis. Awareness and monitored rest are needed. If the symptoms become severe or unmanageable, contact your physician. However, one of the most effective strategies to manage is support. Your support for your loved one and the support you seek for yourself will reduce the stress of the crisis. Support is a buffer against stress and a very important factor during a crisis.

Remember

⇢ **A crisis may cause physical as well as mental changes.**

⇢ **Seek the advice of your physician if the symptoms become unmanageable.**

⇢ **"The experience of grief is not mental illness–it just feels that way sometimes."**
~ Ann Kaiser Sterns

Chapter 3

================

Dealing With Your Own Emotional Pain

"I needed to come to grips with the cancer. I thought the word cancer was an automatic death sentence. I was overwhelmed with the decisions we faced, the quick education we had to get about cancer. At the same time, I appreciated that my wife included me in the process."

~Al Barrineau, support partner

At the time of diagnosis, all attention from the medical staff, family members and friends is obviously directed toward the patient. It is also a very difficult and painful time for you as the person who is closest to the patient. You may be feeling overwhelmed by expectations from yourself and others to be strong and emotionally supportive for your loved one. Recognizing your pain as normal and taking steps to have your own needs met is important. You also need a support system.

You may find that you experience many of the same emotions as your partner–shock, numbness, disbelief, confusion, anger, sadness. All are normal responses. You have also been forced to embrace a dreaded enemy.

This is a sad time for both of you. Grieving is a natural and helpful way for healing to begin. Many find it difficult to openly express these feelings of grief to others for fear that they may appear "weak" or "not in control." The opposite is true. These feelings show that you are very much attuned to what is occurring in your life. Expressing feelings honestly to your partner will not weaken your relationship but will strengthen it. Expressing your feelings to others helps reduce the intensity of the emotion.

Many support partners try to hold back their deep emotional pain and avoid crying. This is not helpful to you or to your partner. Tears do not signal a "loss of control" but more likely convey the intimate love you have for her. Crying is a sign that you are dealing with your emotions in a perfectly healthy and natural way. Seeing your tears will often give her unspoken permission to share her intense feelings and fears.

Gregg Levoy in *Psychology Today* shares, "The amount of manganese stored in the body affects our moods, and the body stores 30 times as much manganese in tears as in blood serum. Biochemist Will Frey says 'the lacrimal gland, which determines the flow of tears, concentrates and removes manganese from the body.' Frey has also identified three other chemicals stored up by stress that are released by crying." Crying is therapeutic.

As the primary support person, you will find it helpful to identify someone you can talk to who understands exactly what you are feeling–a friend, family member or pastor. You also need a support system. Members of a partner's breast cancer support group can assist you in sorting out your emotions. Members have experienced what you are feeling; they understand and identify with you. Talking with someone can serve as a great source of emotional strength during these days.

Cancer treatment centers often offer services such as a partners' support group, social workers, chaplains and counselors who are trained to help you adjust and perform in your new role of support. Remember, you need support, too. You need someone who recognizes the demands placed on a support partner and who can share this experience and understanding with you.

Remember

→ As a support partner, learning to live with someone else's cancer is difficult, but it is a task that can be mastered.

→ Acknowledge your own tears and emotional pain as a normal and helpful response and not as a "weakness."

→ Find someone you can talk to who understands your role of support partner.

It's Okay To Cry

Crying is a very acceptable and healthy expression of grief.
Crying shows how deeply you feel and how much you care.
Crying helps relieve the tension that has built up inside of you.
Crying is an expression of deep contrition and unspeakable love.
Crying speaks for you when you cannot find the words.
Crying helps you to recover your physical and emotional strength.
Crying is not the mark of weakness, but of power.
Crying allows grief to be done in a constructive way.
Crying enables you to cope with a significant loss.
Crying is a way of communicating with your humanity.
Crying ventilates feelings of anger and hurt.

~ Encouragement Ministries

"Tears are salve on our wounds." ~ Nicholas Wolterstroff

*Support Partners
build bridges of hope and
reassurance when others are
vulnerable, exposed and
self-conscious.*

Chapter 4

Understanding the Impact on Your Mate

"My wife told me later that one of the best things I did to help her during those first few days was to cry with her. This seemed to really say to her, 'I'm in this with you. You are not alone.' I knew I had to put her needs first. Listening was important to her. Later I realized this opened the door for good communication for months to come."

~Al Barrineau, support partner

The diagnosis of breast cancer often confirms a woman's greatest fear. With the diagnosis she is thrown into emotional turmoil. She is faced with an array of possible losses or threats:

♦ loss or alteration of a breast
♦ loss of her previous feminine image
♦ threat to her sexuality and attractiveness to you as a partner
♦ threat to her self-esteem because of diagnosis or surgery
♦ loss of her ability to maintain her functional role in the family and/or workplace during surgery or treatments
♦ threat to her life

For a short time following diagnosis, a woman often finds herself in a state of shock and numbness as she sorts through all of these threats and potential losses. At the same time she is struggling to sort out her potential losses, she is expected to make quick, critical decisions–decisions that require a basic knowledge of the disease and her treatment options. This usually leaves her in mental anguish, overwhelmed and with a feeling of extreme loss of control. As a support partner, you can greatly help by understanding her emotional state and by assisting in a manner suitable to her personality and desires.

Creating a Safe Space for Her Emotionally

Most women react to the diagnosis of breast cancer with intense tears and emotional withdrawal. Some find it very difficult to communicate their fears and feelings at this early time. This is all normal. Your partner needs time to grieve over the diagnosis and her loss. Now is the time to give her a "safe space" for her emotions with no judgmental statements, whether you think she is responding appropriately or not. Remember, there is **no right or wrong response** for a woman dealing with initial breast cancer diagnosis.

This is also an extremely hard time for you–particularly the tears, because instinctively you desire to "make things right" and stop the flow of tears. However, tears can be a necessary part of reconciling the loss for many women. Tears are considered a normal, healthy reaction to her diagnosis. Allow her this time and space to experience her emotions in her own way.

As women are groping to understand, most support partners report that they are also hurting and do not know exactly what to do or say. Be assured that no person has been prepared for this time, and everyone searches to understand their new roles of support. It is not easy to deal with your own emotions and try to meet the emotional needs of the one you love at the same time. Occasionally, you may be more acutely and visibly distressed than your partner. This is okay. Remember, people respond differently to a frightening crisis. Individuals have their own characteristic ways of coming to grips with a crisis.

What Most Women Want

When initially diagnosed, women have said that what they needed most at this emotionally distressing time was **not elaborate words or deeds**, but reassurance that their loved one would **be with them throughout the ordeal**. Her greatest need seems to be your **silent presence and assurance that you will be with her through this trial**. Words don't seem to be as important and are often unheard, but your close presence is remembered and appreciated. Try to give her room to grieve in the way she feels necessary without being judgmental. **Don't try to tell her what to do unless she asks.** Assure her of your continued commitment to the relationship.

Anger–A Positive Sign

During the emotionally-charged period following diagnosis, your loved one may display angry outbursts. Loss and fear create anger. Anger needs a target for its expression. This anger may be toward herself for not seeking medical attention earlier or for her non-compliance with screening guidelines. However, more often her anger may be directed at those closest to her. This display usually is not meant to be personal but is an effort to regain control.

Remember, often, in her mind, it is not okay to get angry with her doctors, nurses or God. Therefore, that anger may be displaced onto family members. View her anger as a positive sign that she is not emotionally succumbing to the diagnosis but is beginning to fight back. Forgive her and don't view the bitterness and frustration as directed personally toward you. Don't abandon her physically or emotionally if this occurs. This will all pass.

One woman remarked,

"In my fit of anger and tears at diagnosis I pushed my husband away emotionally. The one thing that happened that made a difference was a note he left reaffirming his love and the fact that this had made him more aware than ever of how important I was to him, and that he would always be here with me. This allowed me to hear what I was afraid to ask. I needed,

*more than anything, to be reassured that this would
not cause me to lose the most important person in my
life; my breast was enough to lose."*

Confirmation of your love and continued presence are the best
responses you can give your partner during the time immediately
following diagnosis. Find your own way to convey your message of
commitment to her during this crisis–tell her, write her notes or show
her by your actions.

Predicting How She Will Respond

Her emotional response now and during the entire experience will
be affected by her personality and prior coping skills. Women respond differently to the diagnosis according to their personalities.
Some women may become hysterical and tearful when they hear the
words, "You have breast cancer." Others, however, may sit staunchly
and show very little emotion in public. Some women want all the
available facts, opinions and information they can gather; others want
only the basic information needed to make a decision. Too much
information can be distressing for some women. Not enough information can be distressing for others.

Some women want their support partner constantly by their side
after diagnosis. Others feel a need to withdraw privately to sort
through their problems on their own. Some want their partner's
verbal input and opinions on treatment options. Others prefer to
make their own decisions. Some want their support partner present
at every office visit or treatment, and still others feel that this is too
emotionally crowding and prefer to go alone unless physically
unable.

Some women find it easy to communicate their emotional pain.
Others find it difficult to express their feelings. Some find looking
at their scar area with their support partners after surgery disturbing
and tend to hide to undress. Others feel very comfortable about
showing their support partners the scar area and openly dress and
undress. **There is no right or wrong reaction**. Each response origi-
nates from complex differences in personalities and is colored by
life's experiences.

A woman will also respond to the breast cancer experience based on the value she places on her breast and her body image as well as on how **she perceives your response**. Age, strangely enough, is not a determining factor of a woman's response to the loss or alteration of a breast. It is a misconception that assumes older women will not be as affected by the impact of surgery as greatly as younger women and are not interested in preserving their body image. This is not true. Some 75 year-old women do not want to have their breast removed and request breast conserving surgery or immediate reconstruction. Personal perception and not age is what determines how women respond.

Some women do not want to leave the hospital after a mastectomy without a temporary prosthesis to camouflage the change in their body image. Oddly enough, some women in their early thirties may request a mastectomy because of their fears of recurrence or radiation therapy, and they place very little emphasis on body image. We cannot predict the value a woman places on her body image or her personal perception of the effects of different treatments.

Pressure from you for one procedure or another can add great stress on your partner. As a support partner, it is helpful for you to learn about the options to be able to discuss them with her. However, it is necessary to allow her to make the final decision and **feel she has your support** for her decision. When women are allowed to take the lead in the decision of how they want their body images preserved or restored after a diagnosis of breast cancer, they seem to make a better adjustment to the procedure and to their new, altered body images.

The best predictor of how your partner will react throughout the breast cancer experience is how she has responded in the past to crises. Take this as your clue as to how she will probably respond and the basis for your support plan. If you are unsure about how she will react, what her needs are or what she expects from you, ask specifically if a certain action will be helpful.

Remember

→ A woman responds to the diagnosis of breast cancer according to her basic personality and previous coping experiences.

→ Response is greatly influenced by her perception of how breast surgery will change her personal body image and how she feels you will respond to the change.

→ There is no right or wrong way to respond to a diagnosis.

→ As a support partner, you need to create a "safe space" for her to work through her emotions.

→ Most women desire your silent, caring presence more than elaborate words or deeds.

→ Perceive anger as a positive sign that she is fighting back rather than succumbing to the diagnosis.

→ Confirmation of your love and continued support is vital.

Chapter 5

===================

What Do I Do First?

"My wife has always coped extremely well during times of crisis. She becomes very organized. She develops a plan of action and puts it into motion. She immediately seeks as much information as she can regarding the crisis. I knew this was one of the first things she needed from me—my help and support as we tried to find out about this enemy that had invaded her body."

~Al Barrineau, support partner

What do you need to do first? One support partner said, "When I heard the words 'breast cancer' from the physician, I felt I had to do everything to protect the one I loved from the hurt. I became mobilized for action. I had to do something. I became very verbal in my opinions as to what she needed to do next on the way home from the physician. The problem came when I took actions which later I found were not needed or appropriate for her diagnosis. I learned I had added much pressure to the pain she was feeling."

As a support partner, you will feel compelled to act to make things better. However, in order to take the appropriate steps, you must allow her time to come to grips with the emotional impact, assess what you can do which will be most helpful to her and then be sure that you both have accurate information before making decisions.

The patient has had no preparation to deal with all of the emotions and complex decision-making demands that accompany the diagnosis. Therefore, as the primary support person, you may be most helpful by locating sources of information specific to her diagnosis. The best source for accurate information is the treatment team. Identify other support persons and someone on the treatment team with whom you can comfortably communicate and who can recommend additional resources.

The overwhelming desire to "make things better" needs to be directed with correct information. Take time to learn the basics of the disease, treatment options and what steps need to be taken in what time frame. Very seldom is breast cancer a medical emergency. Most women have time to learn about their disease and consider various treatment options before submitting to surgery, chemotherapy or radiation treatments.

Usually breast cancer has been in a woman's body for years. A tumor which has a normal growing cycle (doubles every 100 days) and is one centimeter in size (3/8 inch, size of the tip of a woman's smallest finger) could have been in her body for eight years and has just now become detectable. Several more weeks in which to gather information and make educated, appropriate decisions will not adversely affect the outcome for the patient. Women who receive support while reviewing the options, without pressure on specifics from their support partner, will have the foundation needed for emotional recovery.

Remember

→   **Allow her time to absorb the emotional impact. She needs time to cry and express her feelings.**

→   **Obtain correct information from your treatment team before surging ahead with advice or decision-making.**

→   **Assess how you can best help. Resist the urge to rush the patient or to insist on any particular treatment option.**

Chapter 6

Dealing With the Children

"Being open and honest with our children helped us all. My wife had always been there for us. Now it was time for us to be her support and strength. Taking care of Mom helped the boys to deal with their emotions."
~Al Barrineau, support partner

For partners with children the most common question is, "What do we tell the children?" The truth! Children are very perceptive. They know and sense much more than they could ever communicate. They will immediately feel that something is wrong in the family even if you decide not to tell them. What they imagine may be much worse than the truth. From the beginning, it is imperative that you be open and honest with them about what is occurring in the family.

They need to hear the **truth** from you or your partner on a language level they can understand. You do not have to tell everything that is happening, but you need to give them enough information so they will feel a part of the family. Finding out from someone outside the family can weaken a child's trust, resulting in a lowered trust factor in the future.

Tips for telling the children:

◆ If possible, wait until you and your mate have some control of your emotions. For some, this may take a day or two; others may be able to share the first day.

◆ Ask your treatment team for information, or call your local American Cancer Society for information written for children about a parent's cancer.

◆ With your mate, plan what you will say to the children. Plan a time when both of you can share with them and not be interrupted.

◆ Turn off the television and take the telephone off the hook to prevent interruptions.

◆ Start by sharing something similar to the following: "Mommie has found a lump in her breast. The doctor says that the lump is cancer (call it by the right name). Cancer cells grow too fast. The doctor says that he needs to take this lump out because these are not good cells. The doctors and nurses can also help by giving medicine." Continue to share truthfully and simply what the facts are. If you have an example that will explain, this will be helpful.

◆ If you or your mate begins to cry, assure your children that this is because you are sad and it is okay to be sad and to cry.

◆ Allow the children to ask questions. Answer to the best of your ability. If you do not know the answers, be honest and say you do not know.

◆ Reassure them that you will continue to tell them what is happening.

◆ Involve them in the process of helping Mom adjust to surgery and possible treatments. Help them to feel part of the solution to the problem by sharing chores that contribute to the well-being of the family.

Teenage children and grown children also need your open communication and honesty. However, don't be surprised if they don't seem to be overly concerned and quickly return to their normal duties and interests. Take this as a compliment; your openness has restored their confidence that, as a family, you can cope with your new situation.

Families often worry about the effect the illness will have on their children. The most important factor is how you and your mate respond to the illness. If they see you communicating openly, honestly and sharing with a positive attitude, they will more than likely respond the same way. The family can value this time as one of growth and maturity in problem-solving. If you find it difficult to know what to say or realize problems are developing in the family with the children, contact your cancer treatment center and ask for a counselor trained in dealing with children.

In his book, **How Do We Tell The Children?**, David Pertz, M.D., explains:

> *"A child's first question about illness and death is an attempt to gain mastery over frightening images of abandonment, separation, loneliness, pain and bodily damage. If we err on the side of **overprotecting** them from emotional pain and grief with 'kind lies' we risk **weakening** their coping capacities."*

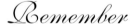

Remember

→ **Children need to be told the truth by you or your partner.**

→ **An illness need not adversely affect children.**

→ **Children usually respond in a manner similar to the way they observe the parents responding.**

→ **A crisis can serve as a time of growth and emotional maturity in a family unit.**

*A Support Partner says,
"We cannot feel the bottom,
but we'll swim until we can!"*

Chapter 7

Dealing With Health Insurance and Employment

"Being properly insured relieved us of one of the biggest problems a lot of people face–the financial responsibility of dealing with a serious illness. We were fortunate. But even if we had no insurance coverage, I would not have let that keep us from getting the medical attention my wife needed. Outstanding bills would have been a small price to pay for her life."
~Al Barrineau, support partner

As you are dealing with the emotionally overwhelming issues of breast cancer, you may find it equally overwhelming to cope with the financial changes incurred by a diagnosis of cancer. Most patients have some form of health insurance coverage to help with the medical expenses. Bills will come from the hospital, physicians, pharmacies, treatment centers, etc. Your challenge is keeping accurate records to ensure optimal reimbursement of claims. This often means constant communication between your insurance carrier and those billing you for service. As a support partner, you can play a vital role by organizing the record keeping; therefore, reducing the stress brought on your partner by the barrage of bills and claims.

If you are insured at the time of diagnosis, call your insurance provider or carefully read your policy for guidelines. You need the following information:

♦ Requirements and procedure for pre-approval for hospital admissions
♦ Requirements for second opinions for surgery or treatment
♦ Guidelines for second opinions from physicians
♦ Procedure to file claims
♦ Claim forms to be mailed to you
♦ Name of person at the insurance company who will handle your claims
♦ Amount of deductibles, if any, before claims are paid
♦ Limits imposed on amounts paid for surgery, chemo - therapy, radiation therapy or reconstructive surgery
♦ Coverage for new or "experimental treatments"–autologous stem cell therapy or autologous bone marrow treatments, etc. may be considered experimental. Ask what they consider experimental and if there are any limits on amounts for such procedures.
♦ Coverage for reconstruction if a permanent prosthesis is purchased (find out if they will pay for both or if one excludes payment for the other).

Keeping up with the filing of claims and payments can become burdensome. However, accurate record-keeping and careful scrutiny of all bills makes the task much simpler. The following suggestions may be helpful:

♦ Purchase a pocket calendar to be used to record all appointments (decide if you or the patient will keep the calendar).
♦ Write on the calendar: physician visits, procedures performed, medication or supplies used.
♦ Provide your physicians with appropriate claim forms and ask if they will file them for you.
♦ Ask for a copy of all charges at the time of service, or ask to have one mailed to you.

♦ Keep copies of all charges from appointments, services, medications or medical supplies in one place (a designated box, file folder or drawer will serve this purpose).

♦ Check periodically to see if appropriate payments are being made to medical providers.

♦ If problems arise with payment, contact your health care facility or provider and ask for help in providing the information needed to receive adequate repayment.

♦ Call your insurance provider and talk with your claims representative to offer additional records or assistance for getting information from your medical providers. (Always record the name of the person to whom you speak. You may need the name for future reference.)

♦ Keep all premiums current. Do not allow your insurance to lapse from lack of payment.

Insurance coverage is more difficult to obtain after any major illness. For this reason be very **careful to keep all premiums current**. Before your partner or you as the primary policy holder decide to change jobs, be sure she will be covered under the new employer's insurance program. If you decide to leave your present employer, ask about continuing your present policy until the new one becomes effective. Many current policies may not cover a pre-existing condition or illness.

Financial Needs

If you realize that this is going to be a financial burden to your family, ask to speak to the social worker in the cancer treatment center. Social workers are trained to help you with the social issues of the illness, including helping you secure financial help for medical services if needed. There are various services available for cancer patients. The earlier you can make this need known, the more effective the social work team can be in helping you. Application for help often requires filing of forms and a period of waiting for approval. People often feel embarrassed to ask for help and postpone the issue. However, many people find that an unexpected illness drains their financial reserves. You are not alone. Ask for help early.

Employment Issues

A woman in treatment will be away from her job for some period of time which varies among patients. Surgery can result in an absence from three to six weeks according to the type of surgery, healing time, and type of employment. Her surgeon will estimate when she is able to return to work. Inform her supervisor of the expected sick leave time that will be necessary following surgery and/or treatment. If treatment is needed after surgery, chemotherapy and radiation side effects vary in patients. The oncologist will need to be consulted as to how much time away from work can be expected. Some women are able to work a normal schedule during treatments. Others have to curtail their activities because of treatment.

Occasionally, a cancer patient may be discriminated against because of illness. However, there are both federal and state laws to protect her. The social worker at the cancer treatment center will be able to help you in this matter. In addition, there are names and telephone numbers of national organizations who deal with these issues listed in the reference section of this book.

Ask your partner what she wants her co-workers and concerned friends to know about her diagnosis and treatment. Some women are very open with their co-workers and friends and talk freely about their disease and its treatment. Other women feel that this is private and desire to keep the details to themselves. Knowing her wishes is helpful because friends and co-workers will come to visit and call to ask about the patient. Being aware of what she wants others to know allows you to answer their questions without invading her privacy. Some women feel it helpful if their support partners communicate with the office during their illnesses, especially during the acute diagnostic period. Patients soon tire of "telling their illness story" and find it a relief to have someone perform this role.

Remember

→ **Wise planning and record-keeping can remove most of the hassle from insurance reimbursements.**

→ **If you need financial help, ask a social worker at your cancer treatment center.**

→ **Support partners can take much stress off the patient by performing record-keeping tasks.**

→ **Ask your partner how much information she would like for her friends or co-workers to know about her illness.**

→ **Issues of discrimination in employment can be brought to the attention of professionals in the area of protection for cancer patients.**

→ **Keep all insurance premiums current.**

*Support Partners
create a safe place for
emotional retreat when
the storms of life threaten.*

Chapter 8

═══════════════

Support Groups

"Getting involved in a support group for mates of breast cancer patients provided a haven for me. I had felt a need to be the strong one for my wife. The support group gave me the opportunity and place to express my concerns, ask my questions, and voice my fears. I was with others who could truly relate to the way I felt: people who understood."
~Al Barrineau, support partner

For some, it may be hard to reach out to others during the breast cancer experience. Often, you doubt if a support group could be very beneficial to you. You may feel you have enough support or could not relate to a support group. However, many find that a support group is one of the most effective methods of management.

Support groups that are disease specific, such as one for breast cancer patients, are composed of people who are going through the same problems of learning to live life under similar circumstances. You and your partner may benefit from a support group. Studies have proven that participating in support groups improves the quality of life and relationships of patients. "Sometimes fear is so engulfing it precludes the ability to call for help," explains one patient. "It is this fear that those of us called patients understand and can help to diminish for one another" (Robert Fisher, Patient To Patient Volunteer Program).

Support groups are a place where people with similar fears and needs meet and share to diminish their anguish and confusion. They are a place where all anxiety, anger and apprehension are understood without any raised eyebrows as to their significance, a place to grow in knowledge and perception of the disease that you are battling. Families and friends are wonderful sources of support, but only someone going through the same life crisis can fully comprehend and empathize. That's the role of support groups. Finding a group for your partner and one for yourself will add a new dimension to your breast cancer experience.

Look for a support group that is led by a professional facilitator who is trained in group dynamics and who knows how to keep the meeting meaningful to those present. A group should offer an opportunity to share experiences, but should not be dominated by "poor me" stories. Instead, educational and support techniques should be provided at each meeting. You may want to talk with the facilitator before attending a meeting to determine if the characteristics of the particular group meet your needs.

For information on breast cancer support groups, contact your cancer treatment center, the local American Cancer Society or the National Alliance of Breast Cancer Organizations. (Addresses and phone numbers are listed in the reference section of this book along with other support and educational resources.)

Remember

→ **For many, support groups offer a safe place to express feelings and receive support.**

→ **Call your American Cancer Society, the National Alliance for Breast Cancer Organizations or your cancer treatment center for names and phone numbers of local breast cancer support groups.**

Chapter 9

Understanding Breast Cancer

"We were shocked and overwhelmed by what we needed to know and what we didn't know about breast cancer."

~Al Barrineau, support partner

Breast cancer is a very complex disease with many variables involved in its treatment. The language and terminology used by the medical profession is often unique to the disease. Therefore, this section is designed to clarify and explain the basic facts of breast cancer in the simplest way.

Cancer begins when the cells in the breast change from normal into cells which have an uncontrolled growth pattern. The cancer cells continue to divide and grow and may spread to other parts of the breast and then to other parts of the body if not removed. The cancer cells can invade neighboring tissues and spread throughout the body, establishing new growths at distant sites, a process called **metastasis**.

Types of Breast Cancer

Approximately 15 different types of breast cancer have been identified. The term **carcinoma** is used by physicians to describe a malignant or cancerous growth. Tumors which develop from different types of breast tissue, in different parts of the breast, may have varying characteristics of development.

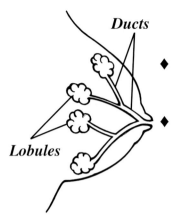

Ducts

Lobules

Breast cancers are named according to the part of the breast in which they develop.

♦ **Ductal carcinomas** begin in the ducts of the breast and comprise the largest number of breast cancers.

♦ **Lobular carcinomas** begin in the lobules of the breast and occur a small percentage of the time.

Ducts or Lobules Cross-Section

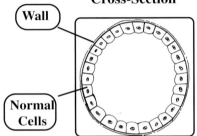

Wall

Normal Cells

Further descriptions of cancers: Normal ducts and lobules are lined with one or more layers of orderly cells.

Normal Cells

♦ **In situ carcinomas** are cancers which are still contained within the walls of the portion of the breast in which they developed; they have not invaded surrounding tissue.

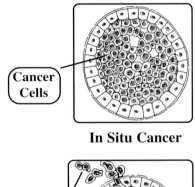

Cancer Cells

In Situ Cancer

♦ **Infiltrating or invasive carcinomas** are cancers that have grown through the cell wall and into surrounding tissues.

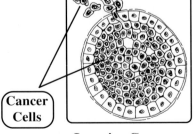

Cancer Cells

Invasive Cancer

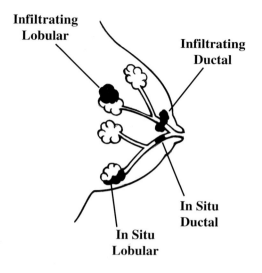

Infiltrating Lobular

Infiltrating Ductal

In Situ Ductal

In Situ Lobular

Growth of Breast Cancer

Some breast cancers grow rapidly, while others grow very slowly. Breast cancers have been shown to double in size every 23 to 209 days. A tumor that doubles every 100 days (the estimated average doubling time) has been in a woman's body approximately eight to ten years when it reaches one centimeter in size (3/8 inch), which is the size of the tip of her smallest finger. The cancer begins with one damaged cell and doubles until it is detected on mammography or by finding a lump. The cancer must be removed from the body using surgery, be killed with either chemotherapy or radiation therapy or be controlled with hormonal therapy. Some believe that cancers may grow in spurts and the doubling time may vary at different times. However, when a one centimeter tumor is found, the tumor has already grown from one cell to approximately 100 billion cells.

Breast cancer is not a sudden occurrence, but is a process which has been developing for a period of time. Therefore, when a biopsy confirms a cancerous breast tumor, your mate is **not facing a medical emergency.** You have time to get answers to your questions and learn about the particular disease and treatment options. Most physicians recommend surgery within several weeks of biopsy. There are exceptions, such as Inflammatory carcinoma (cancer in the lymphatic system), which requires immediate treatment with chemotherapy for maximum control. Ask the physician what recommendations will be made regarding your partner's particular tumor. Tests performed on the tumor will reveal cell type and estimate whether the tumor is a very slow growing or a more rapidly growing tumor.

Some tumors will have the characteristic of spreading more rapidly to other parts of the body. Others do not seem to spread as readily. Breast cancer spreads to other parts of the body through the lymphatic system or the blood system. The spread of the cancer can be local (in the area of the breast), regional (in the nodes or area near the breast) or distant (to other organs of the body). These characteristics will be presented in the pathology report after surgery.

After a biopsy confirming cancer, a woman will usually have to make some decisions about treatment options. These decisions will possibly include surgical procedures, chemotherapy, radiation therapy or hormonal therapy. Surgical decisions will be based on the preliminary (biopsy) study of the tumor.

When the final (surgical) pathology report is evaluated, the oncologist will decide on which treatment is most appropriate for your partner's type of cancer. For some cancers, surgery may be the only treatment needed. Others may require additional treatment with radiation therapy, chemotherapy or hormonal therapy.

Remember

→ **Breast cancer is usually not a medical emergency. You have time to get the answers to your questions.**

→ **The biopsy pathology report is used to make surgical decisions. The final pathology report is used to determine treatment (chemotherapy, radiation or hormonal) decisions.**

Chapter 10

Breast Cancer Decisions

"The best thing our doctors did to help us in the beginning was to keep our primary physician informed. He was the one I looked to, the one I relied on. Their cooperation and good communication were invaluable during our decision-making processes."
~Al Barrineau, support partner

Many women reveal that after they heard their physician say the word "cancer," they remember very little about what was discussed during the remainder of the visit. However, it is essential that information about the extent of the disease and treatment options which are provided in this first meeting be accurately understood. Treatment decisions and necessary action steps are dependent on a complete understanding of what was said by your partner's physician. If you were present when the physician discussed your partner's diagnosis, you can help your partner remember the information relayed. Discuss with your partner what was said to be assured that you both have the same perception.

However, if you feel that you were also overwhelmed and do not have a reliable recall, clarification of information from the physician is necessary. Call your physician to schedule a return visit because this information is vital before treatment options can be explored. Sometimes a period of time, usually overnight, may need to transpire in order for questions to surface that need to be answered.

Often the physician's nurse will be able to answer many of your questions.

If a return call or visit is necessary, be prepared to ask all of the questions that have emerged during your discussions. Take notes or tape-record the answers. You may want to continue the practice of note-taking or recording your consultations with the physician or nurse. In addition, ask for written information on breast cancer, options for surgery and treatment recommendations following surgery. Becoming informed partners with the medical staff is essential in order to regain a sense of control.

Most women eagerly seek help from their partners in gathering information. Occasionally, however, some do not want any intervention past the information gathering stage. They prefer to make treatment decisions completely on their own. Therefore, communication about the desired level of participation between the two of you is crucial if the support is to be helpful to the patient.

The Decision-Making Process

There will be many decisions and conversations with your health care team. Therefore, it will be helpful if you begin to read and acquire a basic understanding of the terminology and types of treatments. Your partner's anxiety level may be so high that she cannot participate in the search for information nor comprehend what she reads or hears. Included at the back of this book is a glossary of basic terms used in the diagnosis and treatment of breast cancer. It will be helpful to familiarize yourself with these terms.

It is very important that the information you collect is specific to her diagnosis. There are approximately 15 types of breast cancer. Furthermore, treatments can vary even with the same type of cancer. Many factors are considered when developing a treatment plan. Ask your partner's physician for the specifics of the diagnosis. Remember, the physician should always be your primary source of information.

The most important questions regarding the specifics of her initial diagnosis are:

♦   What is the type of breast cancer?
♦   What is the size of the tumor?

♦ Is the cancer in situ (inside of the cell walls) or invasive (grown through the cell walls)?
♦ Is there any suspected lymph node involvement?
♦ Is cancer suspected in any other area of the same breast?
♦ Is there evidence that the cancer has spread outside the breast and nodes?
♦ How aggressive (fast growing) is the tumor?

This information will be combined with the age, menopausal status, general health and treatment goals of the patient to help determine treatment recommendations. Before anyone can give you accurate information on suggested treatment, these basic facts will need to be known.

The media–including television, radio and magazines–has taken up the cause of breast cancer education. However, much of this information is very general and may not apply to your partner's diagnosis. The information may be non-approved treatments or may include discoveries unavailable for public use.

Also, be careful of well-meaning friends and their advice. Unless they are professionals in the field of breast cancer, they may offer information which is not applicable and may only confuse you. Remember, the health care team is your best source for accurate advice based on your partner's specific diagnosis and her health status.

If you need more information or clarification on any of the information you read, call the physician's office, cancer treatment center or organizations specializing in cancer. Sources for free information are available from various professional organizations. Listed in the back of this book are names and addresses of these organizations.

Second Opinions

The question of whether a second opinion is needed usually arises. When a medical diagnosis is serious and the suggested therapy difficult to accept, second opinions can serve a valuable role. Surgery, chemotherapy and radiation therapy deserve serious consideration. Accurate and specific information will give you confidence that you are making the best and most informed decisions.

A second opinion is obtained from another physician who practices medicine in the same field. After reviewing all your records, treatment advice will be given. The second opinion can give you reassurance about your treatment decisions. However, for some people, a second opinion may cause anxiety and increase confusion. Some insurance providers require a second opinion before treatment. You will need to check with your insurance company. Physicians may also refer patients for a second opinion to validate treatment decisions. You and your partner should evaluate your needs to determine whether a second opinion will be helpful in your decision-making process.

Reasons for a second opinion may include:

♦   If your mate feels insecure or unsure about what she has been told about treatment options

♦   If your insurance provider requires a second opinion before treatment

♦   If there have been questions or a disagreement within your treatment team about the recommended options for treatment

♦   If your mate wants to learn more about newer therapies not offered by your treatment team

If your mate feels a second opinion would resolve her indecisiveness, ask your treatment team for the name of several physicians qualified in this area. You may also call a major cancer treatment center for a referral. Some centers have multi-disciplinary conferences where a group of physicians from various specialties in breast cancer examine the records, discuss the case and make treatment recommendations.

The most common benefit of a second opinion is to have peace of mind in knowing that all needed information was obtained before a decision was made. An informed decision allows patients to go through treatments confident that they chose the best treatment option for them. If you sense that there are lingering questions or concerns about decisions, encourage your mate to seek a second opinion. These questions or concerns, if not answered to her satisfaction, will often be a source of emotional discomfort in later months. It is helpful to take the time and effort to get answers to her questions now rather than to rush into treatment decisions with a sense of doubt.

Some women feel comfortable with the initial treatment recommendations, feel their questions are answered sufficiently and have no need for a second opinion. This is very acceptable. Seeking a second opinion is an individual decision and one that the patient needs to make according to her needs.

Remember

→ **You must have accurate information on which to make decisions. Only your physician and health care team can provide you with the specifics of your mate's diagnosis.**

→ **Communicate openly with your partner about the extent of your involvement during the decision-making process.**

→ **Request written information.**

→ **Take time to familiarize yourself with the terminology of breast cancer.**

→ **Second opinions may or may not be helpful in the decision-making process.**

*A Support Partner
takes an interest in you
but not a controlling interest.*

Chapter 11

Surgical Decisions

"My wife was not given the choice of surgery options because of her tumor size. In some ways not having to make this decision was easier on us. However, the choice to have reconstructive surgery was not made easily. Helping my wife stand up for what she felt was best for her body took a lot of effort. I'm glad my wife sought my opinion, but the final decision had to be hers."

~Al Barrineau, support partner

Usually, the first decision for the treatment of breast cancer will be the type of surgical procedure to pursue. Breast conserving surgery, commonly referred to as a **lumpectomy**, removes the lump and an area of tissue around the lump. A **mastectomy** removes the entire breast.

Surgical decisions are dependent on many factors including:
- ◆ **Type of tumor** – The type was diagnosed by biopsy and confirmed by the pathology report. There are approximately 15 cell types of breast cancer that vary in characteristics of tumor growth rate and tumor aggressiveness (how likely the tumor may spread to other organs and its potential for occurring in the other breast).

- **Size of the tumor** – Sizes are given in centimeters and millimeters. (Ten millimeters equal one centimeter; one centimeter equals 3/8 inch; one inch equals 2.5 centimeters)
- **Size of the breast** – Some breasts may be too small in comparison to the size of the lump to give good cosmetic appearance when the lump is removed.
- **Location in the breast** – Tumors under the nipple sometimes will not give a suitable cosmetic look when the lump is removed.
- **Possible tumor involvement in lymph nodes**
- **Appearance of mammogram** – To determine if the tumor may be multicentric (occurring in more than one place in the breast). This is sometimes evidenced by microcalcifications (small calcium deposits) or mammographic abnormalities.
- **Involvement of other structures** – The skin, muscle, chest wall, bone or other organs.
- **Patient's desire for reconstruction** – The desired outcome for the reconstructive surgery (breast enlargement, reduction or to match present breast size).
- **General health** – Any treatment limitations due to her present health.
- **Which surgery will give the best chance for a cure.**
- **Which surgery will give the best cosmetic results.**
- **Which surgery will give the best functional results for her arm and shoulder.**
- **Which surgery is associated with the fewest short and long-term complications.**
- **What the patient's priorities are regarding the surgery.**

Each tumor must be evaluated in terms of its unique and specific features and what surgery will be best for the patient. Some types of breast cancer may require chemotherapy treatments before surgery.

Lymph Nodes

During your discussion about breast cancer surgery and treatment, the physician will talk about **lymph nodes**. Lymph nodes are small pea-like structures located very near the breast, under the arm, near the collarbone and near the breastbone. They act as filters for the cells' waste, which is picked up by the lymphatic vessels and filtered through these tiny nodes. Cancer which leaves the breast is often found growing in the lymph nodes near the breast.

Surgeons remove the nodes, and the pathologist (physician who studies cells for disease) evaluates the nodes to see if there is any cancer found. There are three levels of nodes under the arm which drain the majority of the lymphatic fluid from the breast–axillary nodes. These are the nodes that are checked during surgery. The number of lymph nodes removed and evaluated varies according to the type of surgery.

Sentinel Lymph Node Surgery

Sentinel lymph node surgery is a **new** procedure in clinical trials that identifies the first nodes (sentinel) that receive lymphatic fluid from a cancerous tumor, thus identifying the lymphatic drainage pattern. Tumors may drain to different node chains, according to the position of the tumor in the breast. The procedure identifies the chain and the nodes most likely to indicate whether cancer has metastasized to the regional lymph node area. This identification gives the surgeon and pathologist a reliable guide for more accurate node evaluation. Sentinel node surgery **may not** be available in all surgical centers. Ask if it is available in your center.

If available, the procedure is performed when the tumor is removed. The area around the tumor is injected with a radiographic substance and dye several hours before surgery. During surgery, a hand-held gamma-detection probe identifies where the radiographic material has concentrated, and sentinel nodes from this area are removed. After surgery, the pathologist examines these nodes for cancerous cells.

Sentinel node mapping improves the accuracy of selecting nodes to remove surgically and evaluate for spread of the cancer. It may also prevent unnecessary removal of nodes not in the lymphatic drainage field of the tumor. Reducing the number of nodes removed can greatly decrease the potential for lymphedema (a swelling from lymphatic fluid accumulation in the arm which can cause discomfort) and the likelihood of an infection in the arm if any type of injury should occur.

Breast Conserving Surgery (Lumpectomy)

When possible, physicians strive to offer surgery which preserves the body image. However, **breast conserving surgery (lumpectomy) may not be appropriate because of:**

♦   Pregnancy (unless delivery is within six weeks of cancer surgery)

♦   More than one primary tumor in another quadrant of breast

♦   Mammogram revealing suspicious scattered microcalcifications (small calcium deposits seen on film) in another area of breast

♦   Location of tumor in breast (example: located under nipple)

♦   Size of tumor (large tumor or breast too small in relation to size of the tumor will give poor cosmetic results.)

♦   Prior radiation therapy to the breast or chest area

♦   Collagen vascular disease (lupus, scleroderma, etc.)

♦   Severe chronic lung disease (not a candidate for radiation)

♦   Very large pendulous breast (radiation oncologist determines patient's eligibility for radiation therapy)

♦   Evidence of remaining cancer in ducts surrounding tumor after surgery (if surgeon is unable to obtain clear surgical margins, this creates a high risk for recurrence)

♦   Restrictions on travel or transportation to clinic for daily radiation for five to seven weeks

Lumpectomy Procedures

Lumpectomy procedures differ in the amounts of tissue removed based on the size of the tumor. Lymph node removal during breast conserving surgery also varies. Ask the surgeon which of the procedures and the extent of tissue and lymph node removal she will need to have. Listed are the three basic types of breast conserving (lumpectomy) surgeries.

1. Partial or Segmental Mastectomy

The tumor, overlying skin and an area of tissue around the tumor are removed in this surgery. A portion of the lining of the chest muscle under the tumor and some of the skin may also be removed. Lymph nodes may or may not be removed from under the arm by a separate incision, which is approximately two inches in length.

2. Tylectomy

The tumor and a wide area of tissue around the tumor are removed during surgery. Lymph nodes may or may not be removed by a second incision under the arm.

3. Lumpectomy

Lumpectomy removes the tumor and a small wedge of surrounding tissue. Lymph nodes may or may not be removed by a separate incision under the arm.

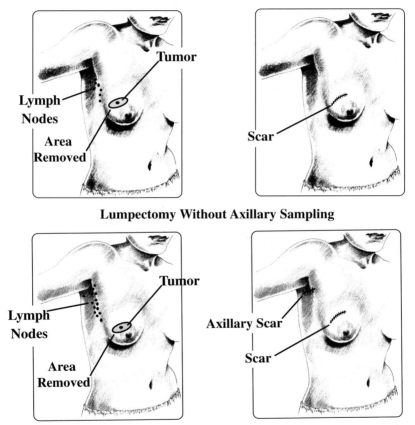

Lumpectomy Without Axillary Sampling

Lumpectomy With Axillary Sampling

Incisions for these three breast conserving procedures are very similar. The cosmetic appearance of the breast after surgery differs only according to the amount of tissue removed.

Mastectomy

There are several types of mastectomies. Your surgeon will tell your partner which procedures will be performed and how much tissue and lymph node removal is planned. The different mastectomies are defined below:

Modified Radical Mastectomy (Conservative or Limited)

A modified radical mastectomy removes the breast, nipple, areola, underarm lymph nodes and the lining over the chest wall muscles.

You may hear the procedure referred to as a "total mastectomy with axillary dissection" which means that the entire breast and some or all of level one and two lymph nodes are removed. The chest muscles and pectoral nerves are not removed.

Full or Complete Modified Radical Mastectomy

A full modified radical mastectomy removes the breast, nipple, areola, **all three** levels of lymph nodes, small chest muscle (pectoralis minor), medial pectoral nerve and the lining over the chest wall muscles.

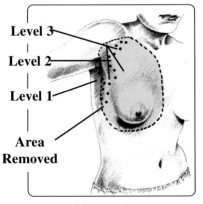

Mastectomy

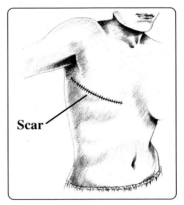

Mastectomy Scar

Total, Simple or Prophylactic Mastectomy

This procedure removes the breast tissue, nipple, areola and possibly some of the underarm lymph nodes that are closest to the breast.

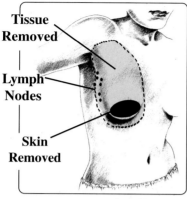

Tissue Removed

Lymph Nodes

Skin Removed

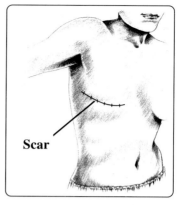

Scar

Simple Mastectomy

Simple Mastectomy Scar

Skin-Sparing Simple Mastectomy

A skin-sparing simple mastectomy is a new procedure used when performing a simple or total mastectomy. The method removes the breast
tissues from a circular incision around the areola (dark colored circle).
The nipple, areola, breast tissues, nodes located near the breast tissues
and additional lymph nodes are removed according to the discretion of
the surgeon. The procedure is often selected when reconstructive surgery
is performed. The sparing of the skin allows reconstructive surgery to be
performed with little need for a period of stretching of the skin. Sensitivity
of the skin over the reconstructed breast remains intact. The reconstructive incision is made using the normal curve of the breast. This incision is
not as visible because it is hidden under the fold of the breast and is concealed by the bra. The incision used to remove the breast is concealed by
the reconstruction of a nipple and areola.

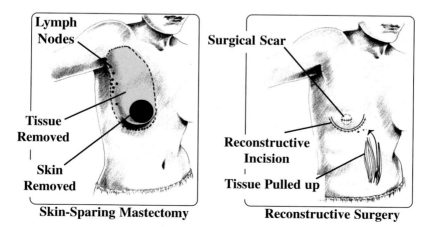

Lymph Nodes

Tissue Removed

Skin Removed

Surgical Scar

Reconstructive Incision

Tissue Pulled up

Skin-Sparing Mastectomy

Reconstructive Surgery

Lumpectomy Versus Mastectomy

If the breast and tumor are within certain size limits, the surgeon may offer your partner the option of a lumpectomy (breast conservation) or a mastectomy. Given this option, the decision may be difficult for her. It needs to be a decision she makes in consultation with her physician, after careful review of the advantages and disadvantages of both. (Remember, the option to choose is not available for some types of cancer.) **It is imperative that she feels comfortable with the decision.** Studies document that a lumpectomy, even if there is local recurrence, **does not affect survival rate.** However, the inconvenience may come from the necessity to have a second surgery. **Note: The surgeon may wish to add additional variables to the following lists.**

Lumpectomy Advantages

- ◆ Preserves body image by saving a large portion of the breast, usually the nipple and areola
- ◆ Patient is able to wear her own bras
- ◆ Slightly shorter hospitalization time, or surgery may be performed as outpatient; shorter recovery time
- ◆ May be psychologically easier to accept unless the fear of monitoring the remaining breast tissue (through breast self-exam, clinical exams and mammorgaphy) is too frightening

Lumpectomy Disadvantages

- ◆ Risk of recurrence of cancer in remaining breast tissue
- ◆ Several weeks, usually five to six, of radiation therapy to the remaining breast tissues
- ◆ Changes in texture, color and sensation of feeling to the breast after radiation therapy
- ◆ Decrease in size of the remaining breast tissues after swelling decreases (following radiation treatments)
- ◆ Monthly breast self-exam becomes more difficult because of increased nodularity (lumpiness) from radiation therapy
- ◆ Possibility of future second lumpectomy or mastectomy if recurrence in breast

Mastectomy Advantages
- ◆ Removes approximately 95 percent of all the breast gland, includes the nipple and areola, thus reducing local recurrence to the lowest degree
- ◆ Reconstruction of breast available using patient's own body tissue or synthetic implants

Mastectomy Disadvantages
- ◆ Body image changed because of the removal of the breast
- ◆ Need for prosthesis or reconstruction to restore body image
- ◆ Recovery time slightly longer than lumpectomy patients

If your partner is having problems deciding between a mastectomy and a lumpectomy, she may wish to speak with patients who have had the procedures. Your physician or your local American Cancer Society's **Reach to Recovery** program coordinator can provide her with a volunteer's name who would be available to discuss her surgical procedure and decision-making experience. When considering a lumpectomy, a consultation with a radiation oncologist to discuss radiation treatments will provide additional insight to make an informed decision.

It is important to remember that a lumpectomy does not affect survival rate, even if there is a recurrence of the cancer. **Each procedure offers an equal opportunity for survival.** The inconvenience is from the possibility of a second surgery if cancer recurs in the same breast.

Reconstructive Surgery

Even though your partner may be losing a breast or a part of a breast through surgery, she has the option to have her body image restored through reconstructive surgery. Breast reconstruction has made a big difference, both physically and emotionally, for many women who have undergone breast cancer surgery. Some women choose to have reconstruction immediately following their initial breast surgery, while others wait until their treatments for breast cancer are completed. Some women choose never to have reconstruction; while others feel that reconstruction will help bring back their feminine silhouette, and they will avoid the necessity of wearing a prosthesis (breast form).

Some support partners are reluctant to discuss reconstructive surgery with their partners for fear of saying the wrong thing or having what they say misinterpreted. Clearly express to your partner that you accept her body image without reconstruction, but that you simply want her to explore any and all options which would be beneficial to her. In order for your partner to be able to maintain a sense of control over the cancer experience, she must be aware of all her options and able to choose those that meet her needs.

Many women have said that their partner's "I want you to do what you need to do" attitude granted them the freedom to discuss reconstruction without the pressure of feeling this procedure was necessary or important to their partner. If your partner expresses any desire to have her body image restored, she should discuss reconstruction with her surgeon **prior** to her breast surgery, thereby preserving all options for future reconstruction. It is also advisable to consult with a reconstructive surgeon prior to surgery, even if she decides to have the procedure performed at a later date. Her surgeon or clinic can recommend reconstructive surgeons.

As with any optional surgical procedure, there are advantages and disadvantages of reconstructive surgery. The decision is to determine if the advantages outweigh the disadvantages. Once a decision has been made to have reconstruction, the next step is for your partner to decide with her physician which type best suits her needs.

The breast may be reconstructed by placing an implant under the chest muscle. Implants may be composed of saline water, synthetic material or a combination of both. Parts of a woman's own body tissue may also be used. This tissue may be removed from her abdomen or back muscle or body fat may be used.

Factors which determine what type of surgery would give the best cosmetic results depend on:
- ◆ Physical makeup (size of breast, degree of sagging)
- ◆ Treatments given for cancer (Prior radiation therapy to the chest area may not allow some types of reconstruction)
- ◆ General health (example: Smokers or diabetics may be poor candidates for some types of surgery.)
- ◆ Desire to enlarge or reduce the other breast during surgery
- ◆ Personal goal and motivation for reconstruction

Age is not a factor for reconstruction. **General health is, however, a primary factor. Health problems that may cause concern and limit surgical options are advanced diabetes mellitus, a recent heart attack or stroke or a history of severe chronic lung disease.** However, only a physician can evaluate the health risks and determine if your partner is a candidate for reconstructive surgery. Some of the advantages and disadvantages of immediate and delayed reconstruction are listed below. Ask your reconstructive surgeon for additional observations.

Advantages of Reconstruction

Retains her feminine body image

Does not have to purchase or wear a prosthesis or special bras

Can wear any clothing, including swimsuits and low-necked attire

Can go braless

Does not have the daily reminder of breast surgery by having to wear a prosthesis

May adjust better psychologically to the disease

Disadvantages of Reconstruction

Physical recovery from surgery will be longer if immediate reconstruction or, if delayed, the need for additional surgery

Expense–some insurance companies may not cover all of the costs, especially surgical repair of the other breast

Increased potential for infection or surgical complications

Immediate Versus Delayed Reconstruction

Advantages of Immediate Reconstruction

One surgical experience, requiring only one anesthesia

Lower cost than two separate surgeries

Reduced recovery time because of only one surgical procedure

Body image not as dramatic or unsettling as from a mastectomy alone without immediate reconstruction

Psychologically, there may be some better adaptation

Disadvantages of Immediate Reconstruction
- ◆ More physical discomfort experienced and longer recovery time following surgery, when anxiety levels are at their highest (surgery time much longer if body tissues are used and only slightly longer if implants are used)
- ◆ Increased potential for infection or surgical complications which could delay treatments

Advantages of Delayed Reconstruction
- ◆ Time to carefully study reconstruction methods and talk to patients who have experienced various procedures
- ◆ Time to carefully select a reconstructive surgeon and seek several consultations if needed
- ◆ Psychologically, less anxiety over cancer experience at time of reconstructive surgery
- ◆ No delay in treatments (chemotherapy or radiation) because of infection or surgical complications from surgery
- ◆ Women with delayed reconstructed breasts may be happier than women who have had immediate reconstruction because they lived with the change brought about by the mastectomy. (They have experienced the inconvenience of having to wear a prosthesis and the constant reminder of their disease; thus, their expectations were not as great as those who chose immediate reconstruction.)

Disadvantages of Delayed Reconstruction
- ◆ Need for a second major surgery
- ◆ Higher cost because of second major surgery (anesthesia, surgery room, etc.)
- ◆ Cost of purchasing a prosthesis and special bras
- ◆ Inconvenience of having to wear a prosthesis until surgery
- ◆ Unable to go braless or wear some low-cut clothing
- ◆ Sufficient time may have lapsed between surgeries meaning insurance deductibles will have to be met for a second time.
- ◆ Psychological distress from having to deal with an altered body image while waiting for reconstructive surgery

Breast Reconstruction Types

Tissue Expander

This is the most common type of reconstructive surgery and provides the greatest flexibility in breast size. The procedure may be done immediately or later as outpatient or inpatient surgery. General anesthesia is usually used and surgery takes from one to two hours to place the expander **under** the skin and muscle. The expander is gradually filled with saline (salt water) solution through a valve every few weeks for several months to stretch the muscle and skin. Additional surgery is required to remove the expander and position the permanent implant.

Implant (fixed volume implant)

A sack filled with silicone gel or saline fluid is implanted under the skin and chest muscle. Surgery is either outpatient or inpatient and lasts from one to two hours. Local or general anesthesia may be used. Silicone gel implants can be used only in clinical trials.

TRAM Flap (tummy tuck)

The **t**ransverse **r**ectus **a**bdominous **m**yocutaneous muscle (major stomach muscle) is moved to the breast area with fat and skin and is attached to form a breast. The transplanted tissue usually remains connected to its blood supply, but occasionally requires microsurgery. Inpatient surgery is required with general anesthesia lasting three to five hours and requiring three to five days of hospitalization. The procedure is moderately painful causing difficulty standing up straight for several days or weeks. A scar is left on the abdomen.

Latissimus dorsi (back flap)

The back muscle, the latissimus dorsi, along with an eye-shaped wedge of skin are moved from the back and sewn in place on the breast area. The transplanted tissues are left attached to their original blood supply. This is an inpatient procedure with general anesthesia lasting two to four hours and requires two to three days hospitalization. The procedure is moderately painful, may require a blood transfusion and a scar is left on the back. Drains may be left in place for several weeks. An implant, in addition to her own tissue, may be required to match opposite breast size. Some procedures can be performed endoscopically (using special instruments under the skin) which does not leave a scar on the back.

Free Flap (microsurgery)

This procedure uses a patient's own tissue from muscles and fat such as buttocks or thighs that are detached (cut free) from their blood supply and reattached to the breast area blood supply using microsurgery. This is an inpatient procedure which includes general anesthesia and may require a blood transfusion. Surgery can range from three to eight hours according to the degree of reattachment necessary. The free flap is the most complex of all reconstructive procedures, requiring a surgeon with expertise in microsurgery. It is moderately painful and there is a longer recovery period.

Nipple and Areola Reconstruction

The nipple and areola are reconstructed from existing skin and fat on the breast itself, or from other areas of the body such as the groin. The skin is molded to form the shape of the nipple and attached to the breast mound. Areola reconstruction may be done by tattooing a dark pigmented color to match the other areola. Surgery is outpatient and pain is minimal.

Women often fear that reconstruction may hide or prevent the detection of cancer recurrence in the breast area. Physicians report, however, that there is little difficulty in detecting early local recurrence because the breast implant is usually placed under the skin and beneath the chest wall muscles. Furthermore, there is no evidence of any kind that breast reconstruction causes cancer to grow or makes it recur. These fears should **not** be of concern in making a decision. Reconstruction may help some women adjust to having breast cancer. For others, it can be an additional stress. Only the patient can make the right decision after she has reviewed all the advantages and disadvantages.

Remember

→ **Surgical and reconstructive decisions need to be made by your partner only, after she understands the advantages and disadvantages of each procedure.**

→ **Encourage your partner to make a decision based on what she feels best meets her needs now.**

Chapter 12

═══════════════

Facing Surgery Together

" My wife is usually the stronger of the two of us, but the day of surgery, she was almost like a child needing her daddy to take care of her–only this time I was the father figure."

～～～～～

"The early morning drive to the hospital was gloomy because of the cold and rain. We were both unusually quiet; each of us was locked in our own thoughts. This was the day we had dreaded, but now that it was here, we were ready to get it behind us. Just as we reached the hospital, the rain stopped and the skies cleared for a short time . . . assurance the sun would shine again for us."

~Al Barrineau, support partner

The period between diagnosis and surgery is an anxious and exhausting time for a woman and her support partner. Before her surgery, the patient will be required to have a **pre-admission assessment** at the hospital or clinic. The physical assessment, which usually takes one to two hours, may include a chest x-ray, blood work, electrocardiogram and instructions for surgery. Though not physically imposing, it is often emotionally distressing and a time most women would find a support partner a comfort. You and your partner should have the following questions answered during this assessment:

♦   What time do we need to arrive?
♦   Where do we park for surgery?
♦   To what area does the patient report?
♦   Should we bring in personal items or wait and take them to the room?
♦   Where will I wait during surgery?
♦   How many people are allowed to wait?
♦   What is the telephone number of the waiting room?
♦   How long is a patient usually in surgery?
♦   How long is a patient usually in recovery?
♦   Who will be relaying information to me concerning her condition?
♦   Will I be able to speak with the surgeon?
♦   What are the visiting hours in the hospital?
♦   Am I allowed to stay in the room overnight if we so choose?

The Night Before Surgery

The night before surgery can be a very sad and stressful event for a woman. This is the last night with her body image intact. Some have to emotionally say good-bye to their breast as if it were an old friend. To ease her distress, plan to make this a special evening for both of you–a quiet early dinner at her favorite restaurant or her favorite food at home. More importantly, however, is letting her know how important she is to you and that you are committed to be with her "no matter what comes." Give her space to work through this time in her own way with your silent support. While women will behave differently immediately prior to surgery, all appreciate a supportive, understanding partner.

The Day of Surgery

You have cried, fought the fears, looked for answers and confronted difficult decisions. On the day of surgery, you both will probably be drained emotionally and physically. However, surgery often brings a sense of relief to the patient, knowing that the enemy has been removed and that she may now go forward.

Allow enough time to arrive at the hospital without rushing. This is undoubtedly an emotional time for both patients and their partners. Most women have a few tears left and are quietly withdrawn and visibly nervous about the surgery. Remember, what most women need is the presence of a support partner. There are no magical words or phrases to erase their fears, but your support will be what makes a difference.

When the patient arrives in her room following surgery, she will be very drowsy from anesthesia. Many women confess that they were not emotionally up to having many visitors the first day. If your partner feels this way, ask the nurse to place a "no visitors" sign on the door so that she can rest and either remove the telephone from the hook or answer the phone for her. Some women feel that this is a very personal time and would rather not have guests until they are feeling more in control of their emotions. Ask her what she would like for you to do to ensure she has adequate rest.

Same-Day Discharge

In some instances, patients are discharged and allowed to go home several hours after they awake from anesthesia. Be sure you understand all discharge instructions before she leaves the hospital or clinic. Read the instructions given to you by her nurse. Ask for any clarification. The patient may be awake and listening but may not remember what is said because of the effects of the anesthesia. Ask for a name and telephone number that you may call if there are additional questions after you arrive home.

You and your partner should have the following questions answered prior to discharge:

♦   How should pain be managed?
♦   What do we do if there is any nausea?

♦   When and what can the patient eat?

♦   When and what regular medications can be resumed?

♦   If she has bulb drain(s) inserted during surgery to remove fluid accumulation at the surgical site, when and how should they be emptied? (Ask for a demonstration.)

♦   Should the amount of drainage be recorded? (Be sure you understand how to measure and record the amount.)

♦   How much can the surgical arm be used?

♦   Does the surgical arm need to be propped up on a pillow while she is lying down?

♦   Should the surgical dressing be changed? (If yes, ask for detailed instructions and for supplies to take home.)

♦   What normal sensations should be expected to occur in the surgical area and arm?

♦   When can a bath be taken? What type of bath?

♦   When can the hair be shampooed?

♦   What symptoms need a physician's immediate attention? (bleeding, increased pain, clogged drains, fever, etc.)

♦   When does an appointment need to be scheduled with the physician? (Do you call for an appointment or has one already been made?)

The Hospitalized Patient

While the time spent in the hospital following surgery is usually short–less than two days–most women have said they appreciate their partner's close presence. "I didn't want him to leave me. . . . Something inside of me wanted to say, 'Hold me and make it all right,'" admitted one patient. Spend as much time as possible with her. She may want you to spend the night with her. While this is not medically necessary, it may be psychologically comforting. Many women need extra closeness. This is the critical time when she needs to know that the change in her body image has not changed your love. Experience reveals that couples who are able to talk openly and assure each other of their committed love will emerge from the breast cancer experience with a stronger relationship.

Getting the Facts

Following surgery, a new set of questions will surface. The best resource for answers is your partner's physician and staff. Most physicians make their daily rounds to patients' rooms early in the morning. If possible, arrange to be in your partner's room at this time to ask the physician your questions. Make a list so you do not forget what you need to ask. If your list of questions will require an extended amount of time to be adequately answered, schedule an appointment with the physician at the office. The nursing staff is also available to answer many of your questions.

Viewing the Scar

> *"I was so grateful a surgical procedure could be performed to rid her body of the cancer. However, my mate had to make peace with her scar before she allowed me to see it. This took several days. We had been able to communicate about it from the beginning and that helped us both. I was prepared for the scar and new body shape to be much worse than it was. I really didn't mind the way she looked. Her breast did not make her the person I loved, and the loss of her breast would not stop my loving her. The scar seemed easier for me to accept than for her–but then, it was her body that was involved and not mine. She needed my assurance that this would not change our relationship."*
>
> ~Al Barrineau, support partner

For some couples, problems may arise when seeing the incisional scar and her new body image for the first time. This event may threaten an intimate relationship more than any other aspect of the breast cancer experience. Some couples recommend viewing the area together the first time, thus avoiding making a decision of when to look. This is usually when the dressing is changed in the hospital or the physician's office. This is never an easy time for the patient or the partner.

Nudity is also a very difficult issue for many women. Those couples that manage best realize that this needs to be faced as early as possible. One woman fondly recalled, "He looked at my scar and said, 'This will always serve as our reminder of how lucky we were to be spared your life. . . . Your breast for your life. Thank God it was a breast, and I still have you. What a deal!' Later, as I looked at my scar, I remembered what he had said, and it was easier for me to accept." Giving special meaning to the new scar early helped this couple avoid a potential problem.

Remember

→ **Accompanying your partner to her pre-admission work-up is psychologically comforting.**

→ **The night before surgery is a highly emotional time for most women. Sensitive planning can make it easier for both of you.**

→ **Most women need extra physical closeness prior to and immediately following surgery.**

→ **Ask for clear discharge instructions.**

→ **Discuss with your partner when to view the surgical area and do not allow it to block an intimate relationship.**

Chapter 13

===

Resuming Communications . . . What Do I Say?

"After surgery she needed to talk and talk. I had never known her to talk so much. She drew comfort from my response, even when it was only a nod of agreement. Listening to her fears, her hopes, and sharing her tears was what she wanted most. At times, I didn't want to hear what she was saying. I wanted to hide in the newspaper or television, but I knew she needed me. I'm glad I took the time to listen."
~Al Barrineau, support partner

Some support partners find it painful to talk about the surgical experience. "Losing my breast was not nearly as hard as losing my mate emotionally. . . . He wouldn't talk about it after surgery," lamented one patient. "He stayed away from home except when he was eating or sleeping. . . . When I tried to talk about my cancer experience, he just looked at me and would not say anything." Communicating after breast surgery can be difficult for both the patient and the partner. Many find it hard to express their thoughts, fearful that they may hurt the other's feelings or emotionally "lose it." Barriers are often erected to prevent this from occurring. The most common is emotional withdrawal–silence.

Emotional seclusion becomes a safe retreat. The workplace or hobby often becomes a safe place to hide. Work absorption becomes the antidote for emotional pain. However, this withdrawal or silence may be perceived as rejection or withdrawal of your love. This may lead to anger from your mate–expressed or internalized–and eventually to depression. This trauma can usually be avoided through early, honest communication. You must talk! You must listen! While painful at first, it is necessary for an emotional recovery from breast cancer. Communicate your feelings to each other–anger, fear, sorrow–whatever they may be. Don't push or force the issue but realize that not talking about cancer may be as dangerous to a relationship as cancer is to the physical body.

Understand that she needs to feel free to express her thoughts without judgment from you. Patients know there are no perfect answers; they just need to talk. Many times women need to say the same thing over and over, so listen. Do not be afraid of her feelings or tears. Tears are a sign that she is in touch with reality and is successfully grieving her loss. Your tears are not a sign of weakness and will not weaken your relationship. "For the first time in my life, I saw the tears in his eyes as we talked about my surgery, and I knew without a doubt that he felt what I was feeling. Somehow from that point on I knew we were going to make it together," shared a patient. Tears have a language of their own and often say what we could never verbalize.

Communicating is difficult for some. They feel they don't know what to say. Spoken under stress, words often become even more powerful and may even be misinterpreted.

In communicating effectively it will be helpful if you **avoid saying the following:**

  ◆   **"Don't worry." "Don't say that."** – This can make your
        mate feel that her feelings are invalid. It will block
        further communication.

  ◆   **"You should . . ." " You shouldn't . . ."** – These words
        strip your partner of her right to take steps to resolve her

own crisis and may cause her to feel a further loss of
control.

♦ **"Everything will be all right."** – An over-generalization
  or an unrealistic view makes a patient's concerns seem
  inappropriate. A better phrase would be "I will be with you
  through this no matter what happens."

Communication Techniques to Enhance Your Relationship:

♦ **Solicit information:** "Tell me how you feel about . . . "
  "Share your thoughts about this decision with me." – This
  allows doors of communication to be opened. Some
  women need verbal permission to share.

♦ **Non-verbal:** Instead of words, use your body language to
  speak. Hold her hand; make eye contact; place your hand
  on her shoulder; sit or lie close to her; lean forward when
  she is speaking; wink at her when you catch her eye in
  public. A large part of communication is body language.
  Your body language can be a very powerful source of
  comfort and communication. It can convey your love and
  concern.

♦ **Restate her words:** "I hear you say you need/want . . ."
  "I understand you would like to . . . " – Restating clarifies
   to your partner that you hear her requests and feelings.

♦ **Observe her body language:** Observe her frowns, ques-
  tioning stares or tears. "I feel that you may be tired . . .
  upset . . . concerned . . . confused about. . . . Is this an
  accurate observance?" Observing her body language and
  verbalizing these observations conveys absolute recognition
  of her needs and then allows her to verify or communicate
  previously unspoken concerns.

♦ **Ask for her input:** "I need help in determining what to tell
  the children/family/friends." "How do you want me to
  schedule help with the housework."– Asking for her input
  in decisions allows her to remain a viable decision-maker
  in the family and reassures her of your need for her continued partnership.

Effective communication with your partner is one of the best tools for recovery. Direct, sensitive communication between partners in a caring non-judgmental manner facilitates a healthy acceptance and problem-solving approach.

Remember

✦ **Communication is even more essential after breast cancer.**

✦ **Women listen intently to what you say and observe your body language. Be careful not to send mixed messages.**

✦ **Listening is an important part of communications. Let her talk. Talking can be therapeutic.**

"The art of communicating is not only saying the right thing at the right time, but also leaving unsaid the wrong thing at a tempting moment."

Chapter 14

Understanding the Pathology Report

(Detailed Study of the Tumor)

"In the beginning, I thought my wife would die. I thought breast cancer was a death sentence. When the physician explained the particulars of her pathology report, it gave us renewed hope that our dreams for the future could still be realities. We were told the factors that were significant for her prognosis. Several things in the pathology report helped us know that her cancer was part of a large disease, but was also uniquely hers. We could draw strength from others, but we could not make comparisons."
~Al Barrineau, support partner

Most treatment decisions will be based on information from the biopsy and surgical pathology reports, taking into consideration her age, menopausal status, and general health. Pathology reports are often very technical and difficult for a lay person to understand. Yet, the pathology report contains most of the vital information on which treatment decisions are based. Years ago, pathology reports were kept secret from patients and their families. Today, many physicians feel it is helpful if patients and their families understand the diagnosis to the degree with which they feel comfortable. The pathology report may help a patient understand why a particular treatment protocol is needed and why it may be unlike someone else's they know. This is often accomplished by the physician's explanation of what the report reveals. Because this explanation may be hard to understand without a lay interpretation of the meaning of the terms used, it is included in this book.

You may find it helpful to familiarize yourself with the terms you may hear during discussions about treatment decisions. **While it is not essential that you or your partner understand all of the following information**, you may find it helpful as a future reference if needed. Some pathologists are happy to explain the report.

There will be two pathology reports. The first will be from the biopsy and the second from the surgery. Surgical decisions are based upon the preliminary biopsy report, which is combined with the final surgical pathology report to determine stage and need for further treatments.

How the Tumor Is Assessed

When the tumor is removed from the breast, it is sent to a pathology laboratory. There, a pathologist, a physician who specializes in diagnosing diseases from tissue samples, analyzes and issues a pathology report to your physician. This report will help the physicians determine if additional treatment is needed. If additional treatment is needed, the pathology report will be used by the oncologist (cancer specialist) to develop a treatment plan for the patient's cancer, based on the findings in the report. The report will give information on the following aspects of the tumor:

Common Types of Breast Cancer

- ♦ Infiltrating or invasive ductal (approximately 54%)
- ♦ In situ ductal or intraductal (approximately 19%)
- ♦ Invasive or infiltrating lobular (approximately 5%)
- ♦ In situ or noninvasive lobular (approximately 2%)
- ♦ Medullary (approximately 6%)
- ♦ Mucinous or colloid (approximately 3%)
- ♦ Paget's disease, intraductal or in situ (approximately 1%)
- ♦ Paget's disease, invasive or infiltrating (approximately 1%)
- ♦ Cancers occurring in 1% or fewer patients: Tubular, Papillary, Adenocystic, Inflammatory, Scirrhous, Apocrine, Squamous.

There are various other rare types of breast cancer and combinations of the above types.

Tumor Size

Tumor size is the largest dimension of the tumor. Results are reported in centimeters (cm) or millimeters (mm).

      10 mm equal 1 cm.

      1 cm equals 3/8 inch.

      1 inch equals 2.5 cm.

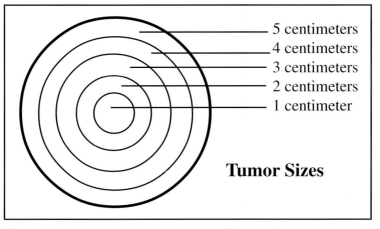

5 centimeters
4 centimeters
3 centimeters
2 centimeters
1 centimeter

Tumor Sizes

Margins

Margins describe the area surrounding the tumor, or if the entire tumor was removed, it is how the margins relate to the tumor. If the tissue surrounding the tumor had **no** evidence of cancer cells, the terms used will be "clear," "clean" or "uninvolved." If cancer is found in the margins the terms may be "involved," or "residual cancer." It the pathologist is unable to make a definite statement the term "indeterminate" may be used.

Shape

The report may also state the shape of the tumor as round or spherical (well-circumscribed) or an irregular shape (stellate, poorly circumscribed). The more irregular the shape of a tumor, the higher the potential to be aggressive.

Characteristics of Cancer

The cancer will either be in situ or invasive. (Illustration page 30)

    ◆   **In Situ Cancer** – Normal ducts and lobules are lined with one or more layers of cells in an orderly pattern. It is considered "in situ cancer" when cancer develops and grows but does **not** break through the wall where it began and remains in the duct or lobule.

♦ **Invasive (Infiltrating) Cancer** – Cancers that have broken through the wall of the duct or lobule and have begun to grow into surrounding tissues in the breast are called invasive or infiltrating.

Node Status

If surgery included lymph node removal, the report will state how many nodes were removed, a description of the area from which nodes came and how many nodes tested positive with cancer cells.

Grading of Tumor

The grading of cells is a microscopic examination describing the degree of change from the original, parent cell. This grading determines aggressiveness. Tumors are classified as:

♦ **Grade 1: Well differentiated tumors**—Less than 25% of cells are abnormal. Approximately 75% or more of the cells are very similar in appearance to the parent cell from which they evolved. They look similar, like sisters. Usually least aggressive.

♦ **Grade 2: Moderately differentiated tumors**—About 25 - 50% of cells are abnormal. Between 50 - 75% of cells still resemble the parent cell. They are like first cousins. Term describes cells between the well and poorly differentiated stages.

♦ **Grade 3: Poorly differentiated cells**—Nearly 50 - 75% of cells are abnormal; 25 - 50% of cells resemble the parent cell. Similar to third cousins. Usually aggressive.

♦ **Grade 4: Undifferentiated cells**—More than 75% of the cells are abnormal. Only 25% or less of the cells in the tumor are normal. These cells do not resemble any family member. Usually most aggressive.

Scarff/Bloom/Richardson Tumor Grading Scale

Some pathologists use the Scarff/Bloom/Richardson grading scale. This grading system gives a number from 1 to 3 according to aggressiveness of three different characteristics: 1- tubular formation, 2- nuclear size and shape, 3 - mitotic count. The numbers from each characteristic are then totaled to determine the aggressiveness of a tumor. The higher the number, the more aggressive are the characteristics of the tumor.

Characteristics Evaluated Using the Scarff/Bloom/Richardson

Evaluates cell arrangements for characteristics of looking like a small tube.

1. Tubular Formation	Grade Value
Majority >75%	1
Moderate degree 10 - 75%	2
Little or none	3

Evaluates size and shape variation of cells and nucleus of cells.

2. Nuclear Shape/Size	Grade Value
Uniform nuclear shapes	1
Moderate increase in varying shapes	2
Marked variation (often large nucleus)	3

Determines how many cells are visible in the dividing stage in an area of the tumor.

3. Cell Division Rate	Grade Value
Low (0-5)	1
Moderate degree (6-10)	2
High (>11)	3

Total of the scores in the above three areas of evaluation determines final grade.

Final Cumulative Total	Points
Grade 1 - well differentiated	3-5 points
Grade 2 - moderately differentiated	6-7 points
Grade 3 - poorly differentiated	8-9 points

A higher final Scarff/Bloom/Richardson score indicates a more aggressive tumor.

Prognostic Indicators Other Than Grade

◆ **Necrosis** (cell death) may be noted in a report. Cell death is a result of the lack of necessary oxygen and nutrients to parts of a tumor causing the cell to die. This signifies a more aggressive cancer. Often necrosis is related to a comedo (type of aggressive cell) component.

◆ **Blood Vessel (Vascular) or Lymphatic Invasion**
A microscopic examination of the tumor will show if the surrounding blood vessels or lymphatic vessels have been invaded by the tumor. No invasion offers a better prognosis.

Prognostic Tests

Various tests may be ordered to look at specific characteristics of the tumor cells.

♦ **DNA Status:** A test that looks at the genetic material found in the DNA (blueprint for cell reproduction) of a cell. Normal DNA of a cell appears with two sets of chromosomes. **DNA ploidy** determines DNA composition of cells. Tumors may be:
• **Diploid** means having two sets of chromosomes, which is normal.
• **Aneuploid** refers to the characteristic of having either fewer than or more than two sets of chromosomes; this is abnormal, suggesting aggression.

♦ **DNA index** is the ratio of aneuploid DNA compared to diploid DNA.

Proliferation Markers

♦ **S Phase Fraction** – Flow cytometry reveals number of dividing cells and corresponds to the growth rate of a tumor.

♦ **Mitotic Rate** – Microscopic observation of number of cells that are dividing.

♦ **Ki67 Stain** – Microscopic observation of all dividing cells. Increase in any of the above proliferation markers suggests an aggressive tumor.

Hormone Receptor Assay

A hormone receptor assay is a chemical or observation test that measures the presence of **estrogen** and **progesterone receptors** in the tumor cells. It tells the physician whether the tumor was stimulated to grow by female hormones and is very important in determining what type of treatment will be used. If a tumor is positive, that means it was stimulated by estrogen or progesterone and usually carries a slight increase in a positive prognosis. Positive receptor tumors may be treated with anti-hormonal medications such as (Tamoxifen) for control.

Tumors may be: ER+ (positive) and PR+ (positive)
ER- (negative) and PR+ (positive)
ER+ (positive) and PR- (negative)
ER- (negative) and PR- (negative)

HER-2/neu Oncogene

HER-2/neu (c-erbB-2) oncogene is a substance in cells that promotes tumor development. This oncogene is found amplified and over-expressed in about 20-30% of breast cancers. Recently it has been demonstrated that HER-2/neu over-expression can predict the response to Adriamycin-based chemotherapy, as well as resistance to Tamoxifen. Furthermore, the recent introduction of immunotherapy with a "humanized" monoclonal antibody, Transmuxtab (Herceptin™) directed at the HER-2/neu protein, has required further screening of breast cancers for HER-2/neu over-expression to determine if these types of drugs may be effective.

There are many other diagnostic tests being used to evaluate tumors. Your physician will discuss with you the tests selected to evaluate your tumor. Each of these tests helps collect pieces of the puzzle needed for the oncologist to determine your best treatment.

The pathologist prepares a written report that is sent to your physician. Time varies as to when the final report will be available. Check with your physician on how long your laboratory requires. After reviewing the pathology report, your physician will decide if further diagnostic tests, such as a bone scan, liver scan, chest x-ray, CT scan or an MRI (magnetic resonance imager), may be needed to stage your cancer.

When all the results are received from the tests, your partner's cancer will be **staged** on a scale from zero (in situ cancer) to four (a cancer with distant metastasis). A stage zero cancer is the earliest with the best prognosis. Staging is an estimate of how much the cancer has already spread and is important in selecting appropriate treatment.

Three basic factors are considered in staging:
 ◆   tumor size
 ◆   lymph node involvement
 ◆   metastasis to other areas

Stage 0

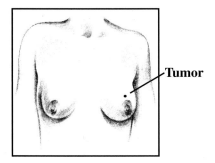

Tumor in situ (inside duct or lobules); negative nodes

Stage I

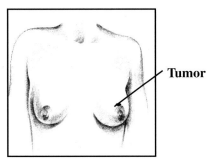

Tumor confined to breast, 2 cm or smaller; negative nodes

Stage II

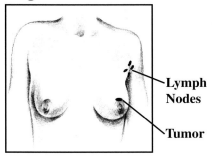

Tumor 2-5 cm; movable positive axillary nodes; or tumor over 5 cm with negative nodes

Stage III

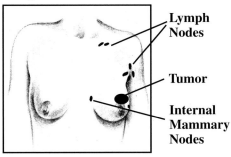

Tumor over 5 cm with positive nodes; or involvement of skin, fixed axillary nodes or internal mammary nodes

Stage IV

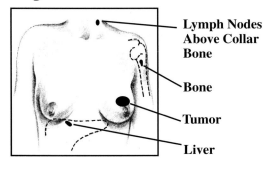

Distant metastasis to other parts of the body. Examples illustrated are the liver, bone and lymph nodes above the collar bone. Cancer may have spread to other sites or a combination of sites in the body.

When your partner returns to the physician for her pathology results, she may want to ask the following questions and write down the answers. Some doctors will provide a copy of the pathology report for her records, and some pathologists will discuss the report with the patient.

Questions to ask about the pathology report:

What is the name of the type of cancer?

Was the tumor in situ (inside ducts) or infiltrating (invasive, grown through the cell walls)?

What size was the tumor? (The size is in centimeters or millimeters.)

Was the cancer found anywhere else in the breast tissue? (The term **multifocal** means additional cancer was found in the same quadrant as the tumor; **multicentric** means it was found in another quadrant of the breast distant from the tumor.)

How many lymph nodes were removed? How many levels of lymph nodes did you sample or remove? (There are three levels of axillary nodes.)

Were any lymph nodes positive with cancer cells?

♦ Were the tumor receptors estrogen or progesterone positive or negative?

♦ Was the tumor HER-2/neu positive or negative?

Was the cancer diploid (like a normal, original cell) or aneuploid (unlike normal cells)?

What was the S phase, mitotic index or proliferative status (how fast cancer is/was growing)?

Is there anything else we need to know about her cancer?

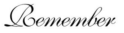

Remember

↦ **The pathology report contains information needed to determine treatment decisions.**

↦ **Individuals must decide how much they wish to understand about cancer. As a support partner, it is most helpful if you assist her in getting and understanding the pathology report to the degree that she feels comfortable.**

*Support Partners
keep each other from bolting,
fleeing in panic and emotionally
retreating when the storm clouds
loom on the horizon.*

Chapter 15

===================

Treatments for Breast Cancer

"As a little league football coach, I learned that the first step to winning is to build a good team. I thought about this when my mate faced a breast cancer diagnosis. If we were to win this game, we needed the best team. Our family doctor acted as head coach, my wife became the quarterback, and, at times, I only felt like the water boy; but, by putting together the best medical and supportive team we could, we knew we were doing all that was humanly possible to give her the best chance for recovery."

~Al Barrineau, support partner

After the final pathology report is studied, the oncologist (physician who treats cancer) will recommend a plan of treatment. This may include chemotherapy (treatment with cancer-fighting drugs), radiation therapy (x-ray) or hormonal therapy. Some women will receive all these treatment methods. Others may only receive one type of treatment. Some women may not receive any treatment because of their tumor characteristics and the surgery performed.

Treatment decisions are made by an oncologist. The oncologist will carefully review the pathology report and any other tests, perform a thorough physical exam and then prescribe a treatment plan.

This treatment plan will be designed according to:
- cancer cell type
- size of tumor
- in situ or invasive cancer
- growth rate of tumor
- evidence of spread of cancer to other parts of the body
- lymph node involvement
- how much the cells had changed from original cells
- estrogen and progesterone hormone receptor status
- menopausal state of the patient
- medical history
- general health

Remember, there is more than one kind of breast cancer, and different types of cancers may require different treatment. Some types of cancer, and cancer that has spread to other parts of the body, **may** require chemotherapy administration **before surgery** is performed. **Do not compare treatment with another patient's treatment** because you will probably be comparing two altogether different cases.

Chemotherapy

Chemotherapy drugs are usually given into a vein, but, occasionally, they are administered by pill. Treatments usually consist of a combination of several drugs. Treatments usually begin several weeks past final surgery and are given in a clinic or physician's office. Frequency of administration varies according to the treatment plan and is usually completed in four to six months. Side effects vary according to the drugs, amount of drugs administered and the individual patient. The treatment team will supply information on the drugs and management of side effects.

Some women with poor veins may require a permanent device inserted under the skin called a venous access device or a "port" ("port-a-cath"). This device is usually placed under the skin on the chest wall and is used to administer chemotherapy and draw blood samples. The patient is able to perform normal activities with the device, including bathing and swimming.

For cancer that has spread outside of the breast or a very aggressive tumor, your partner's physician may suggest bone marrow transplant or autologous stem cell transplant. These treatments are usually performed in cancer centers. Numerous guidelines and criteria regarding age, extent of disease and prior treatment are considered in the recommendation of these therapies. If recommended, ask for written information.

Radiation Therapy

Radiation therapy is used after a lumpectomy or for local control when cancer has spread into an area. Therapy is delivered to the area to kill remaining cancer cells by a machine that produces high energy x-rays from radioactive substances. Treatment usually begins when the incision has healed–four to six weeks. Each treatment only takes minutes after the initial visit and is given on a daily basis, Monday through Friday. Side effects may include changes in the skin over the treated area, mild fatigue and, occasionally, a sore throat.

Hormonal Therapy

Hormonal therapy may be recommended if the studies performed on the tumor prove to be estrogen or progesterone positive. The most commonly used drug is Nolvadex® (tamoxifen citrate tablets). While doctors don't know exactly how Nolvadex® works, they acknowledge that it blocks the effects of estrogen on breast cancer cells. It does not kill but may control remaining cancer cells that may have been left in the body after surgery. It does not cause the side effects of chemotherapy. There is no hair loss or fatigue.

Nolvadex® is given by mouth once or twice a day. The most frequently reported side effects are hot flashes (80% on Nolvadex®, and 68% on placebo) and vaginal discharge (55% on Nolvadex®, 35% on placebo). In studies with Nolvadex® the risk of cancer of the lining of the uterus or for blood clots in the lungs and legs increased 2 - 3 times compared to placebo, although occurring in less than 1% of women. Women who have a history of blood clots or who require anticoagulant medication should not take Nolvadex® for risk reduction of breast cancer. Stroke, cataracts and cataract surgery also occur more frequently with Nolvadex® therapy. In addition, if your partner is prescribed Nolvadex® and is premenopausal and sexually active, it will be necessary to ask the physician about appropriate nonhormonal birth control. Women who are pregnant or expect to become pregnant should not take Nolvadex®.

Breast Cancer Genetic Testing

In 1994 and 1995 two mutated (changed) genes, BRCA1 and BRCA2 (BR=breast, CA=cancer), were discovered that cause 7 - 10 percent of breast cancers. A blood test can now determine if a person is a carrier of either mutated gene and the possible cause of her breast cancer.

After a breast cancer diagnosis, the health care team can review the patient's family and personal history to determine if she meets the criteria for genetic testing. Genetic testing can determine if she has a mutation in either of these identified genes. If positive, her children, male and female, are at a fifty percent risk of inheriting these defective genes, placing them at higher risk for breast, ovarian or other cancers. Testing consists of having several tablespoons of blood drawn and sent to a laboratory.

Who Is A Candidate For Genetic Testing?

- Person with breast and/or ovarian cancer who has **two or more 1st or 2nd degree** blood relatives (on either the mother's or father's side) with either breast or ovarian cancer
- Person with breast and/or ovarian cancer who has a **1st or 2nd degree** blood relative who was diagnosed with breast cancer **under 45** (or premenopausal) or a relative who has ovarian cancer **at any age**
- Personal history of breast and/or ovarian cancer **before age 45**
- Personal history of breast and/or ovarian cancer that is bilateral (both sides) or with multiple primary sites
- Males who develop breast cancer
- Person who has a 1st or 2nd degree relative with a positive gene

Benefits of BRCA1 and BRCA2 Genetic Testing:

- Allows you to know if cancer was related to one of these mutated genes
- A negative test might prevent unnecessary anxiety about your children being high risk and prevent future expensive surveillance tests
- Allows family members to choose to be tested or placed in high-risk surveillance programs if patient has an identified positive gene

Remember

➥ **Treatment for breast cancer is based on the pathology report and the individual characteristics of the patient.**
➥ **Chemotherapy, radiation therapy or hormonal therapy may be prescribed.**

Chapter 16

Your Partnership in Recovery

*"The one I loved most was battling for her life.
We were in this together."*
~Al Barrineau, support partner

The chronic phase of recovery for the patient, partner and family begins when the patient returns home. The acute emotions of the diagnosis slip into the background while the conflict of merging new family roles with the old routines–meals, cleaning, laundry, jobs, school–becomes the focus. The patient often struggles with the realization that she may no longer physically maintain her role in the family. Change becomes difficult as your family life takes on a lower emotional tone and concentrates on reassigning chores of daily living. As a mate, you will strengthen your family relationship by becoming a part of the solution to the routine chores.

Look for opportunities to help in her physical as well as emotional recovery. When your partner returns home, she will probably need to have her dressing changed and her drain bulbs emptied. Some women appreciate assistance, while others feel uncomfortable. Ask her how you and the family can be more helpful. The surgeon will instruct your partner on when to begin an exercise program that will help her regain strength and mobility in her surgical arm. One patient's support partner became the "captain of her physical therapy team."

The partner reminded her of her exercises and helped her perform them. By participating with her in the dull, routine exercise series, this partner restored a vital sense of caring in the patient's mind. This teamwork kept them emotionally in touch during a time of physical readjustment for both of them.

Support During Treatments

> *"I do not like hospitals. I do not like being around sick people. But the person I loved most in the world was having to have chemotherapy treatments in our fight to save her life. I was glad to go with her."*
> ~Al Barrineau, support partner

Chemotherapy or radiation treatments may be required after surgery (see Chapter 15 on chemotherapy). The time of treatments can be very anxiety-provoking for your partner. While she will probably be physically able to go for her treatments alone, psychologically she may need someone to accompany her, especially on the first visits. A support person–you, a family member or friend–can help relieve her anxiety and help her understand the oncologist's explanations about her treatments. Your mate may be hesitant to ask for you to go with her, but she will be very grateful when you offer to go or find someone else to accompany her. Others may not want "so much fuss" made over their treatments and will feel more in control if they go alone when they are physically able. Communicating your willingness and desire to share this time is important to her.

Planning to be helpful during treatments begins by understanding what her treatments involve. Your oncologist and staff will answer the following questions to help you and your partner plan and adjust during chemotherapy and/or radiation treatments:

   ◆   How often will treatments be administered?
   ◆   How long will each treatment session last?
   ◆   Is someone allowed to be with the patient during these treatments?

◆   What are the expected side effects of the treatment and when do they occur?

◆   Will any medication which could prevent her from driving be given prior to or after treatments?

◆   At what time during the treatment cycle will she become the most fatigued?

◆   Are there any side effects, signs or symptoms which need to be recognized and reported to the health care team?

By understanding these facts you will be able to make this time as psychologically and physically comfortable as possible. Plan to have food available around treatment dates so she will not feel responsible for meals. She may wish to schedule treatments to be given on Fridays, so you may take over household responsibilities over the weekend, allowing her plenty of time to rest. One couple made a ritual of renting several movies and made this their weekend to catch up on their movie watching. The children pulled their sleeping bags into the den, and everyone "camped out" around Mom. The weekend was eagerly anticipated instead of dreaded, despite the physical discomfort experienced by the patient. Carefully assess her physical and psychological needs so you may be as supportive as possible during treatment.

Treatments may physically drain and fatigue the patient, resulting in her inability to resume her prior life-style and routines. Her daily responsibilities may have to be redistributed among family members, co-workers and friends. One husband told of his experience taking on unaccustomed chores. "I already did most of the cooking, but I learned to do the laundry, only ruining a few items as I learned. We had a cleaning person come in one day a week on a regular basis. The expense was not too great and was certainly worth the energy it saved. Ideally, I wanted the kids to do more; however, they are normal and haven't become much more useful around the house." Recognize the need for changes–household chores, family, work, community activities. Take the initiative in reassigning responsibilities and helping your mate prioritize her duties during recovery.

Understanding the Side Effects of Chemotherapy on the Relationship

Chemotherapy treatments may impact a relationship both physically and mentally. You will receive much information on how to manage physical side effects such as nausea, diarrhea, low white blood counts and the resulting fatigue. In addition, medications and helpful interventions will be provided by your oncologist. However, several other side effects–fatigue, hair loss and sexuality changes–may profoundly impact your relationship, requiring special understanding and support from you.

Hair Loss–The Most Painful Side Effect

> *"When my wife lost her hair during chemotherapy treatments, it was almost the proverbial 'straw that broke the camel's back.' Losing her hair seemed to strip her of the last defense she had in denial of her own cancer."*
> ~Al Barrineau, support partner

Many women have expressed that losing their hair through chemotherapy treatments was one of the most distressing of all losses during breast cancer. Even though the hair loss is temporary and will return after treatment is completed, its impact is described by women as "being as upsetting as the loss of my breast." Hair loss is difficult because it is outward evidence of the cancer process. It is often the first visible public display of their battles with cancer. It is much easier to camouflage the loss of a breast under clothing than the loss of hair with a wig.

The amount and timing of hair loss will vary according to the kind of drugs, the dosage of the drugs and the individual response to the drugs given. Most hair loss occurs between two and four weeks after the first treatment. Some treatment regimens will only cause gradual hair thinning; others will cause complete hair loss. To help you and your partner prepare for this occurrence in the treatment process, discuss with the treatment team how much hair loss to expect and when it may occur.

To help your partner deal with her hair loss, discuss what you have learned and assure her of your total acceptance. It is recommended that she shop for a wig before she loses her hair to better match her hair color and style. Her wig will probably not be noticeable except to those who know she has lost her hair. Do not complain about the cost of wigs or insist on her getting one which she does not feel comfortable wearing. She needs your support and understanding during this extremely sensitive time.

Obviously, the day or week she loses her hair will be one of her lowest emotional times. You can't change it. You can't make things different. Your best response is your reassuring presence. Allow her to grieve her loss and shed her tears as she feels necessary.

Many people revert to jokes and humor during uncomfortable and painful times. However, support partners advise against using nicknames such as "Baldie," "Kojack" or other terms denoting hair loss. She may laugh outwardly but may inwardly feel different. Let her take the lead in how she can best react and manage her new appearance. Respect her privacy as she dresses and undresses. It is usually much more difficult to allow you to see her bald head than to let you see her scar. Remember, hair loss is usually temporary. Therefore, don't insist that she show you her bald or thinning head. This will pass, unlike the change in her body image.

Some women will cling to the security of their wigs after their hair begins to return. She may need your encouragement to shed the wig and show off her new, shorter haircut. For some, this takes courage because they may have entered treatment with longer hair and may only feel comfortable returning to that image. This can be especially difficult if they feel that longer hair was important to you. Let her know of your acceptance early in the treatment phase.

Effects on Your Sexual Relationship

> *"We were both emotionally drained. I had to give my mate a chance to regroup. The actual sexual act could wait. However, we both needed touching, cuddling and holding each other. It was important that I tell her I still found her attractive. I allowed her to set the guidelines on how and when the sexual relationship would be resumed."*
>
> ~Al Barrineau, support partner

You may notice your sexual relationship changing during the recovery period. Obviously, her energy level will be low, and she will not feel like doing much of anything. She may be physically and emotionally exhausted. This is all temporary. A danger exists only if these changes are misunderstood by you and your partner.

Most women have expressed that they really needed and wanted more touching, hugging and emotional closeness. But they didn't know how to express this or were afraid to ask. You may also feel unsure in your response and find yourself withdrawing as well. Do not allow walls of silence and emotional isolation to separate you from your partner and diminish your sexual relationship. Let her know you still desire to be close and touch without sexual expectations or demands.

Chemotherapy treatments cause a reduction in the amount of female hormones in the body. As a result of this hormonal change, women may experience symptoms that mimic menopause, such as lessening of normal sexual drive, vaginal dryness and mood changes. By understanding these changes and their causes, your relationship with your partner should not suffer but thrive.

While a reduced sex drive may exist, this does not mean that it is absent. Sexual arousal may just take longer. Therefore, partners need to look for innovative ways to stimulate each other in a patient, caring way.

Hormonal changes cause the vagina to have less lubrication resulting in vaginal dryness. The vagina will take longer to lubricate during sexual arousal. If not understood or corrected, these problems can result in painful intercourse and possibly a small amount of bleeding. Supplemental hormones are not recommended. However, there are over-the-counter vaginal lubricants in the pharmacy (Replens® or Vagisil®)designed to maintain the moisture in the vagina. These are applied **inside** the vagina on a **regular basis**, several times a week, to restore and hold moisture. They are **not** designed as a lubricant before intercourse. Before intercourse generously apply a liberal amount of a lubricant (Astroglide®, highly recommended by patients, or K-Y Jelly® but **not** Vaseline®–which can promote vaginal infections) and reapply as needed.

Not only can vaginal dryness be uncomfortable; it can also set up an environment for irritating or painful vaginal infections, in addition to interfering with sexual pleasure. If any itching or swelling is experienced, the patient should contact her physician for evaluation for a vaginal infection. Infections are often caused by an overgrowth of fungus normally found in the body. This can be easily treated with medication. Ask the physician if treatment is also recommended for you, the sexual partner, as well as for the patient.

It is almost a certainty that mood changes will occur during treatments. The reduction of the female hormones caused by treatment may cause wide fluctuations in her moods. She may swing from normal to sad, to angry, to depressed, all with no apparent cause. It is important to understand that she, like you, dislikes the changes she experiences. Relating to her mood swings in an understanding manner, realizing the cause and not interpreting this as a sign of a diminishing relationship, is important.

However, what will change is how she feels about herself and how she views her attractiveness as a sexual partner. You must let her hear and be assured that her reshaped body image has not changed how you see her–that her true beauty, sexuality and attractiveness are just as strong for you now as they were before her surgery. This is essential for the normal resumption of the sexual relationship.

Although it may sound silly, it is important to know that cancer cannot be "caught" from a partner during the sexual relationship. There is no reason that a sexual relationship should not continue in the same manner as before the cancer diagnosis.

If no complications arise, the incision should heal in about four weeks following surgery. The area will still be tender but should not be painful. You may resume your sexual relationship before the area is totally healed. The best time to continue, however, is when both of you, as partners, feel ready.

Tips for resuming the sexual relationship:
- ◆ Communicate your continued attraction to her as a sexual partner. Find as many ways as possible to convey this message. Say it. Write notes. Send cards. Touch her.
- ◆ View the incision area soon after surgery and get this major obstacle to sexual functioning out of the way.
- ◆ Verbalize your desire for the resumption of the relationship.
- ◆ Prepare for sexual relations by having adequate amounts of a water-based lubricant available if needed.
- ◆ Plan a time when her energy is at its highest.
- ◆ Plan a special time for closeness–a special date, dinner, movie or whatever she enjoys.
- ◆ Plan a special time to touch and stroke her body. Sexual arousal will be slower and foreplay may need to be longer because of the reduction of female hormones.
- ◆ Don't force or ask her to remove her gown or prosthesis if she does not feel comfortable. This may cause her to emotionally withdraw. Some women said that it took several months before they really felt free to participate in intercourse without their scar area covered. Others admitted never wanting to have sexual intercourse without their scar area covered, even though the partner had seen the incision. Do what she feels is comfortable and what does not reduce her sexual feelings.
- ◆ After intercourse, remain close and continue to touch her in a loving way. Assure her that she is still the same loving partner and gives you the same pleasure.

As in all other areas of the breast cancer experience, women and their partners will react differently to each situation. Use these tips as suggestions only. Some partners have said that their sexual relationships were even more gratifying after the cancer experience.

Recognizing and understanding that changes following surgery and treatments are a normal and temporary part of the recovery process will make you a more sensitive partner. If problems do arise at a later date and you have difficulty working through the changes, trained sexuality counselors are available in most cancer treatment centers.

Remember

→   **Surgery and treatments can cause physical changes which you need to understand.**

→   **Hair loss can be the most traumatic of all events for a breast cancer patient.**

→   **Changes in sexual functioning can be caused by side effects of treatment.**

→   **Resumption of the sexual relationship needs to be approached with sensitivity and planning.**

→   **Birth control should be discussed with the physician.**

*Support Partners
remain by your side no matter
how deep the waters of
adversity rise.*

Chapter 17

Her Emotional Adjustment
to Breast Cancer

"Breast cancer threatened our relationship. We are taking advantage of our second chance. We've fallen in love all over again. I've seen my wife blossom before my eyes."

~Al Barrineau, support partner

Breast cancer can serve as a "wake-up call" to life. In one woman's words, "I realized that I was not going to live forever when I received my diagnosis. I had never stopped to think about it! But now I live every day to the fullest. No longer will I be a slave to those things in life that were of no consequence." A new lease on life, a desire to make every day and minute count, is often the result of the cancer experience.

A year after her surgery one patient reminisces, "Breast cancer was the worst thing that ever happened to me and the best thing that ever happened to me. Even though I hated every change my cancer caused my family to go through, as I reflect, it has brought us a greater degree of happiness and love, and today I would not trade the experience." Many patients and families report a greater degree of happiness after breast cancer because they decided to concentrate on happiness rather than things. Facing the dreaded enemy caused them to refocus their priorities.

This is an excellent time to encourage your mate to do some things she has always wanted to do but did not take the time for. Encourage her to use breast cancer as the reason to do the things she dreams of and not as an excuse not to. Support her in beginning a hobby, taking a class, getting a pet, planting a flower garden, planning a trip–whatever she has an interest in doing. A sense of accomplishment will provide a helpful environment for emotional and physical recovery.

When Adjustment Becomes Difficult

> *"My wife had a history of clinical depression so we had an added area of concern as to how she would handle all of this. She did great in the beginning, but, after chemotherapy, a new kind of tears and withdrawal started. We then tried one-to-one counseling and a breast cancer support group. Encouraging, talking with, crying with and receiving encouragement from others walking in the same shoes helped her tremendously."*
> ~Al Barrineau, support partner

By the time most women complete their treatments they have adjusted emotionally to the experience and are putting their lives back to a normal routine. Occasionally, someone has difficulty returning to normal. If the one you love has problems, you will need to alert someone on the health care team. Being the person closest to the patient, you will be able to accurately recognize if your mate is continuing to have problems coping. If this should occur, inform your primary care physician.

Often, patients do not consider their mood disturbances a concern that they should take to the physician. They sometimes think that **continuing sad feelings are normal, but they are not.** As a support partner, your close relationship to the patient allows an understanding of what is normal behavior for the patient and what is not. The first step is to understand how to distinguish a **normal reactive depression** from a **clinical depression.**

Distinguishing Normal Depression From Clinical Depression

Normal depression after a loss is an expected reaction. It is described as "feeling blue or feeling down." This usually means that the person may feel sad but can still enjoy and look forward to parts of her life, such as a family gathering, a movie or seeing a friend. Clinical depression is severe depression that causes many physical and emotional changes and needs the intervention of a professional. Clinical depression is often manifested by:

- Continuous feeling of sadness (not several days but weeks)
- Social withdrawal from family and friends
- Feelings of worthlessness
- Excessive feelings of guilt
- Excessive feelings of fearfulness
- Feelings of hopelessness
- Being very slow in physical movement or speech
- Feeling constantly jittery or nervous
- Low energy level; may feel tired all the time
- Inability to make decisions
- Negative thinking
- Imaginary health problems
- Lack of interest in food or eating excessively
- Disinterest in work or day-to-day activities
- Uninterested in intimacy or sex
- Insomnia (inability to sleep–wakes early or cannot go to sleep) or sleeps too much
- Suicidal thoughts*

*Immediately notify a health care professional of suicidal expressions or threats.

If your partner exhibits several (some say five or more) of these symptoms for a period of two weeks or longer, your physician should be notified.

Treatment of Depression

Depression may be treated in several ways. In some cases, counseling may be all that is needed. Counseling identifies weakness in coping skills and works to strengthen them. Often, talking to an understanding person accomplishes much for a depressed person.

However, medication may be needed to assist the process. Antidepressants are often prescribed and will take approximately two weeks to become effective. Diet and exercise have also been proven to be beneficial to reduce depression and stress. Ask your physician for recommendations.

It is important that your mate understands that **depression is not a sign of weakness.** It is a legitimate condition that is experienced by many people after a major crisis or loss. Most depression is periodic, and short-term counseling and medication will help through this period of adjustment. Identifying and seeking help is the first step to resolving the problem of depression. If you feel that this may be occurring in your partner, **encourage her to call her physician. If the depression is severe, you may have to notify her physician.** She may lack the emotional energy to reach out for help.

Events Which Trigger Normal Reactive Depression

Post-Treatment Depression

After a major loss, there are periods of normal depression which may be predicted. There is a period of depression that often occurs–several weeks after or at the end of treatment–when the patient is no longer going to the cancer treatment center on a regular, monthly basis.

One patient recalled, "Somehow I felt while I was getting chemotherapy that they were doing something about my cancer; then all of a sudden I completed my treatments. I thought that this was the time that I had waited for so intensely over the past six months, but to my surprise, I felt frightened. No one was doing anything. I was not seeing anyone. Then the fears overwhelmed me. I didn't know if I could make it on my own. I found myself experiencing many of the sad feelings I had felt at diagnosis, the tears started back . . . I withdrew emotionally, my appetite left, and I was unable to sleep. But, thankfully, a family member brought my condition to the attention of my physician. I was relieved to know that these feelings happened to many patients at the conclusion of their treatments, and, after talking openly with them, I began to understand."

The conclusion of chemotherapy or radiation therapy treatments is a common time for patients to experience depression. The months of constant contact with the health care staff provide a sense of security and socialization for the patient. When treatment ceases and her medical support system is not present, she becomes very concerned and may feel somewhat alone. Periods of sadness exhibited by the patient are normal and sometimes last for several consecutive days. But, if this time turns into weeks, it is advisable to seek assistance for the loved one.

Anniversary Depression

Another common time for depression is around the anniversary date of her diagnosis, surgery or other events surrounding the cancer diagnosis. These dates may serve as triggers for an "anniversary reaction" and result in a short period of depression. The date brings back all the memories of the event so clearly that the patient finds herself reliving the event to the point that many of the old feelings return. The result may be a brief period of depression.

One psychiatrist, who had bilateral mastectomies, plans a special event for herself on the day of her original diagnosis for breast cancer. She plans a light work day or, if possible, takes the day off and treats herself. She plans for family members or friends to spend this time with her. Wise planning can help during these expected times of emotional conflict. Yearly regression into many of the old, experienced feelings may happen for years after the event. This is a normal reaction to a traumatic event. Careful planning around these dates to avoid further stress, in addition to your understanding, will help during this time.

Physical Checkup Depression

Return visits to the physician for checkups can also renew many of the anxious, depressed feelings associated with breast cancer. Many women experience high levels of anxiety for several days surrounding their return visits to the physician for checkups. Know that this reaction is normal and allow her these brief periods of emotional regression. Check to see if she needs you to be with her for these checkups. If so, plan to accompany her or arrange to have a friend or family member go with her to the physician.

When Treatments End

The breast cancer experience will have changed many things for you and for your mate. Understanding and recognizing some of the major emotional traps of post-treatment depression, anniversary reactions and return physician visits will allow the two of you to plan wisely to maneuver through the emotional storms.

By the time surgery, treatments and reconstruction (if chosen) are completed, you will have been under extended stress. Do not be surprised to find yourself suffering from exhaustion when it is all over. This is a time to plan something special for the two of you to enjoy together. It is also the time you will need to find out what schedule of tests and visits will monitor her health in the future. Mark your calendar and then try to put breast cancer out of your focus for a while.

Remember

→ **Normal (reactive) depression is expected after a major loss.**

→ **Support partners can learn to recognize clinical depression, which needs the attention of a health professional.**

→ **Depression usually responds to intervention with counseling and medications.**

→ **Anniversary dates, treatment completion and return office visits can cause a reactive depression which may last for several days. Wise planning and support can help reduce the extent of the reaction.**

→ **Plan a special treat after surgery and treatments end. You deserve it!**

Chapter 18

Managing the Fear of Recurrence

"Surgery, chemotherapy and reconstruction were all behind us. Yet, there was a cloud of fear over our lives– recurrence. Finding the proper balance between necessary follow-up care and obsession with recurrence can prove a challenge especially the first few years. The new appreciation for each other and life itself will be lost if you don't control and deal with your fears."

~Al Barrineau, support partner

At a time when the battle with treatment for breast cancer is over and life can resume some sense of normalcy, the fear of recurrence can serve as a dark, black cloud. This fear can rob couples of a sense of safety and pose a great obstacle for happiness, adding much stress to the relationship. This fear was the most often expressed fear by support partners of the patients I worked with in support groups.

To gain a sense of control over the fear of recurrence, it will be helpful if you take steps of management. The first step is to acknowledge your fear. The second step is to know that your mate has the same fear. She, too, has to deal this joy robber of the future. It will be very helpful if you can face this obstacle as a team. Talking with each other about the need to rationally approach the problem will be a foundation for your plan.

How do you manage the fear of recurrence as a couple? Denial is certainly not the answer. Understand that this is the most common fear of support partners. It is a natural fear. You are completely normal to feel this fear, as is your partner. In fact, for couples who do not experience this anxiety, there is a danger that they are not dealing with the reality of a breast cancer diagnosis. No one can ever guarantee anyone that there is no more cancer in the future. The greatest problem I have encountered is the fact that most couples do not have an accurate understanding of the realistic risks of recurrence. More often, their fears are exaggerated far greater than the truth.

There are guidelines, however, that can help predict the risks of recurrence. You need to know these risks. This is the first step to managing fear–accurate information. To begin with truth, you and your mate will need to talk with her physician. You cannot manage what you don't know. This information must come from your mate's health care team and not from the media or well-meaning friends. Accurate information is necessary.

Management Strategies for Fear of Recurrence:

Make an appointment with your physician to talk about your mate's particular risks. Some mates feel a need to talk to the physician in private about their partner's risks. You will need to decide what will best meet your needs. Ask the following questions:

1. What are her risks for recurrence?

Most often, the risk is overestimated by support partners. You need to know the truth. But, remember to use statistical data as guidelines and not fact. Every woman is an individual and does not necessarily fit the statistical tables.

2. How often will she return to you for a checkup?

Return visits for checkups vary. They are usually every three months after treatment and are gradually reduced if no problems arise.

3. What diagnostic tests do you plan to perform on these checkups?

Bloodwork and a physical exam are performed on each visit. Physicians have various schedules on which to perform mammograms, bone scans, liver scans, CT scans, chest x-rays, etc. Ask what scheduled tests are planned as follow-up care. Women are often frightened when they are scheduled for some diagnostic tests. They think the physician is suspecting recurrence, when in reality the test is a regularly-scheduled follow-up test for all patients.

4. What signs and symptoms do we need to report?

Your physician will tell you the most likely signs of recurrence, according to the type of breast cancer your mate had. Cancers vary in their likelihood of recurring in a specific manner. Your physician can help you know which symptoms need immediate medical attention.

5. What can we do to maximize her recovery?

Ask about diet, exercise, breast self-exam and medications she should or should not take (example, estrogen-type mediations). Physicians will often recommend professionals to work with the patient to learn about diet, exercise programs and breast self-exam. Encourage your mate to participate in learning, but do not force her. Patients often need a time for emotional retreat and find it stressful to take on any new challenges.

One of the ways you may help is to offer to participate in some of these recovery strategies. You may both wish to change your dietary habits or start an exercise program together. Breast self-exam is also a necessary tool to help monitor for recurrence in the remaining breast and the scar area. Women report that this often causes much stress and they are often fearful to perform their exams. One way you may help is to offer to learn to do the exam for her. One husband reported that his wife was overwhelmed with fear about checking her breasts. "I asked for instructions and I now perform this task for her monthly. . . . It is not a bad job! . . . . In fact, this has been our bonding time in fighting the fear of recurrence together." Look for your own ways to make recovery a partnership.

6. Whom should we ask to speak to if we have questions?

Most physicians have a nurse who is qualified to answer many questions by patients and to refer those that need a physician's attention. Identify this person. It is normal to think that every pain is a sign of recurrence the first few years. Managing these fears is best accomplished by communicating with the appropriate person who can appropriately evaluate your concerns. Utilize this fear management technique. If you have any questions call and refer the questions you have to this person immediately, rather than resorting to worry. Use your health care team as your referee as to whether there is a cause for concern.

Open the Door for Communications:

The next step after accurate information from your health care team will be the need to build an open, honest relationship with your mate. She needs to feel that she can share her physical concerns and fears without "upsetting" you. Women often feel uncomfortable sharing physical symptoms; they don't want to worry anyone. However, you can help monitor her health, if she feels free to tell you how she is feeling or any physical changes occurring.

As we discussed previously, she also needs to have freedom to verbalize her fears in times in which she is vulnerable—checkups, anniversary dates and times of depression. Her road to recovery may have some detours of anxiety. This is normal. You can help by recognizing these times, allowing her to talk and giving her support.

One of these fearful times is checkup visits. Checkups are a very anxiety-provoking occasion for most women. Ask if she would like to have you accompany her to the physician. Your presence may be very helpful. Help her plan a stress-free schedule, if possible, around anniversary dates of diagnosis or surgery. She will vividly remember these dates and your acknowledgment by being supportive will be very helpful to her emotional recovery. Plan a special treat—a meal out, a single flower, a note telling her of your love—to make these times easier. **Remember, she is not looking to you for miracles, only your understanding and support.**

We have been discussing managing fears of recurrence as partners and how you can help your mate by allowing open communication. Yet, a very vital part of your personal fear management is finding someone with whom you can openly share of your fears and feelings. This will be found in support groups, friends, professional counselors, and spiritual counselors. Look for these sources of support from those who truly understand and avail yourself of the help they offer. One support partner said, "We need to understand the needs of our mates, but we also need to understand and meet our own needs for support. I found this source in a support group of other mates. That is when I finally managed to get my fears under control. . . . I needed support too."

"To fight fear, ACT. To increase fear—wait, put off, postpone."
                                        ~ David Joseph Schwartz

"Fear is conquered by action. When we challenge our fears, we defeat them. When we grapple with our difficulties, they lose their hold upon us. When we dare to face the things which scare us, we open the door to freedom."
                                        ~ Wynn Adams

"You gain strength, courage, and confidence by every experience in which you really stop to look fear in the face. The danger lies in refusing to face the fear, in not daring to come to grips with it. You must do something you think you cannot do."
                                        ~ Eleanor Roosevelt

Remember

→ The cloud of fear of recurrence is a joy robber, and it must be addressed with accurate information and open communication for optimal emotional recovery by you and your mate.

→ Accurate information is obtained by consulting with the health care team concerning risks and signs and symptoms which need to be reported.

→ Mates have predictable times when their fears of recurrence increase—physical checkups and anniversary dates. Wise planning can reduce the intensity of their fear.

→ Mates need to feel free to express their fears and physical symptoms with you without upsetting you. This allows you to monitor her emotional and physical recovery.

→ You, too, need support partners. Reach out to those who can best meet your need by understanding your fears and offering support when you are vulnerable.

→ Mates are not looking to you for miracles, only loving support.

Chapter 19

═══════════════

Shared Insights on Coping

"Finding the proper balance in your life is a challenge, especially in the first few years after diagnosis. The new appreciation for each other and life itself will be lost if you don't control your own fears. Take interest in her emotional as well as physical recovery; but do the same for yourself. You aren't going to be much help to her if you don't take care of yourself."

~Al Barrineau, support partner

Working as a Breast Cancer Specialist, I had the opportunity to observe hundreds of mates as they worked through the breast cancer experience with the ones they loved. It is not an easy task. Being a support partner is one of the most difficult tasks because there is no training and there are very few guidelines to allow you to know if you are doing the right things.

My observations reveal that some partners become so hyper-vigilant in their new role that they forget to take care of their own needs as they endeavor to meet all of their mate's physical and emotional needs. Some feel inadequate and fail to try to make things better. They fall into a pattern of denial or avoidance of their mate's crisis and leave the patient to depend on friends or other family members for support. Most often, mates muster all of the emotional muscle available and learn to become the support partner needed by the patient.

In this effort, I have seen wonderful things happen to couples. I have seen relationships grow into a deeper commitment. I have witnessed a new love develop for the partner. One patient shares, "We feel like we did when we were dating 25 years ago. We can't wait to see each other at the close of the day. Somehow we had gotten so busy we had lost each other in a flurry of careers and activities. Breast cancer gave us back the gift of our love for each other." Many relationships experience this renewal.

Working closely with mates in support groups and as individuals, I had the privilege of listening as they shared the things that made a difference in helping them in this new role as support partner. I asked support partners to share with me their best advice in our effort to make your journey a little easier.

- ♦ Acknowledge your mate's and your own emotions. Don't stifle them. Don't try to be too positive; this can be as difficult for your mate as your being depressed.

- ♦ Find someone you can trust–someone who understands your needs–and talk with them. We all need support; it makes life easier to bear.

- ♦ Gather up-to-date information on the disease and become knowledgeable of the basic decisions that need to be made. Often women are paralyzed with fear and cannot take these steps. Knowledge increases your sense of control and allows you to become partners with the health care team.

- ♦ Recruit needed help from your family and friends. They want to be helpful and appreciate it when you tell them specifically what your needs are at the time.

- ♦ Keep organized in your record-keeping. Get a calendar and keep records of appointment dates and treatments received. Ask for copies of bills to file for future reference. This will help when insurance companies and hospitals are billing you for services–often months later.

- ♦ Rearrange your previous priorities, realizing it will be for a limited period of time, not forever. A golf game may need to be exchanged for a walk with your mate or an outing to the mall for her emotional support. You may even need to

take an occasional "mental health" day from work to take
care of your own emotional and physical needs.

♦   Plan special and fun times for you and your mate together.
Often, recreation and fun times are abandoned during
treatment, but this should not be the case. Be creative in
how recreation may have to be changed because of limited
amounts of energy, but plan some time of diversion for the
two of you.

♦   Seek feedback from your mate. There is a careful balance
between communication and silence, withdrawal and over-
involvement, separateness and togetherness, attentiveness
and emotional distance. Mates have different involvement
needs. Be sure that you are not extending too much energy
in areas that she may feel are unnecessary.

♦   Take care of yourself physically. As your focus changes to
your mate's needs during surgery and treatment, be sure
that you remember to watch your diet and eat regular,
balanced meals; avoid overeating or skipping meals; get an
adequate amount of sleep; avoid alcohol, smoking or drug
use (these will lower your resistance physically); and
maintain some type of exercise. Exercise is one of the best
ways to reduce stress. Walk with your mate, ride bikes
with the children or go to the gym. This will relieve much
tension.

♦   Add the magic. Say, "I love you," often, and be as creative
as possible in conveying the message. One couple shares,
"Breast cancer gave us the opportunity to fall in love all
over again." Use this time as an opportunity to rekindle
your relationship.

One support partner expressed, "Today, I am a different person. I
know what pain of the heart feels like, and, from knowing pain
personally, I have grown into a stronger, more sensitive and
compassionate person–a person I like better."

Remember

→   **Breast cancer is not a planned event in the lives of couples. Yet, in the crisis are the seeds for the growth and strengthening of the relationship as you help the one you love face this enemy.**

→   **"We cannot tell what may happen to us in the strange medley of life. But we can decide what happens in us and how we take it, what we do with it, and that is what really counts in the end. How to take the raw stuff of life and make it a thing of worth and beauty . . . that is the test of living."**

~Joseph Fort Newton

"At diagnosis I thought we were given a death sentence. Today, I know that doesn't have to be the case. With the right medical team, educating yourself about cancer and faith, there can be a better quality of life after breast cancer.

Harriett now serves as a Reach To Recovery Volunteer visiting, educating and encouraging newly diagnosed patients as they begin their new battle with breast cancer. I gladly share my experiences with new support partners.

We don't take each other for granted anymore. We now have a regular habit of dating–another good thing that came out of the experience. Our relationship has priority.

*As I look back, I can honestly say that, as bad as the breast cancer experience was for both of us, it has resulted in tremendous growth as individuals and as a couple. **It can do the same for you."***

~Al Barrineau, support partner

Resource List

National Alliance of Breast Cancer Organizations (NABCO)
NABCO is a nonprofit national central resource for information about breast cancer and acts as an advocate for breast cancer patients' and survivors' legislative and regulatory concerns. For more information write to NABCO, 9 East 37th Street, 10th Floor, New York, NY 10016, (212) 889-0606 or fax (212) 689-1213.

AMC Cancer Research Center's Cancer Information Line
Professional cancer counselors offer easy-to-understand answers to questions about cancer, provide advice and support and will mail instructive free publications upon request. Equipped for deaf and hearing-impaired callers. Call (800) 525-3777.

American Cancer Society.
A toll-free hotline provides information on all forms of cancer and referrals for the **Reach To Recovery** program for breast cancer patients which provides a visit by a peer who has had a similar type of surgery. Call (800) 227-2345.

The Komen Alliance
The Komen Alliance is a comprehensive program for the research, education, diagnosis and treatment of breast disease. Write to The Susan Komen Foundation, Occidental Tower, 5005 LBJ Freeway, Suite 370, Dallas, TX 75244, or call (212) 450-1777 or (800) I'M AWARE.

The National Coalition for Cancer Survivorship
The National Coalition for Cancer Survivorship is a national network of independent groups and individuals concerned with survivorship and sources of support for cancer patients and their families. NCCS is a clearinghouse of information and advocates for cancer survivors. Write to NCCS, 1010 Wayne Ave, 5th Floor, Silver Spring, MD 20910 or call (301) 650-8868.

Physician Data Query
PDQ is an arm of the National Cancer Institute that provides accurate information to patients, care givers and doctors through a computer. Information about cancer treatments and clinical trials that are open to patients is available. Names of organizations and doctors involved with cancer care can also be obtained. Call (800) 4 CANCER for details.

Y-Me National Breast Cancer Organization
Y-Me provides support and counseling through their national toll-free hotline, (800) 221-2141, available 24 hours. Write to 212 W. Van Buren, Chicago, IL 60607.

Insurance or Legal Matters

The National Insurance Consumer Helpline
A hotline established to answer consumer questions and provide problem-solving support and printed materials for patients. Lines are manned by trained personnel and licensed agents and are available 8:00 a.m. to 8:00 p.m. Eastern Standard Time, Monday through Friday. Call (800) 942-4242.

National Insurance Consumer Organization
Organized to educate consumers about their insurance rights through publications and telephone inquiries. Call (202) 547-6426 or fax (202) 547-6427.

American Cancer Society
Cancer: Your Job, Insurance and the Law (4585-PS)
Summarizes cancer patients' legal rights regarding insurance and employment; gives complaint procedure instructions. Call (800) ACS-2345.

The Americans With Disabilities Act: Protection for Cancer Patients Against Employment Discrimination (4585, 1993)
This brochure defines the ADA law by describing employment rights of the cancer patient.
Call (800) ACS-2345.

The Consumer's Guide To Health Insurance (C103)
The Consumer's Guide To Long-Term Care Insurance (C101)
*The Consumer's Guide to Medicare Supplement Insurance (*C101)
These are guides prepared to help the patient understand health insurance coverage. Call (800) 942-4242.

SUGGESTED READING:
Man To Man, by Andy Murcia and Bob Stewart. New York: St. Martin's Press, 1989. This book was written by two men after their wives had surgery and treatment for breast cancer. This is an honest, in-depth look at the emotions and physical changes that occur in the family unit during the breast cancer experience. This book is available at your local bookstore in paperback for approximately $11.00.

References

Arnold, Elizabeth, and Kathleen Boggs. **Interpersonal Relationships.** Philadelphia, PA: W.B. Saunders, 1995.

Bland, Kirby I. **The Breast 2nd Edition**. Philadelphia, PA: W.B. Saunders Company, 1998.

Bohmert, Heinz H., and Patrick Henry Leis, Jr. **Breast Cancer**. New York, NY: Thieme Medical, 1989.

Casciato, Dennis A., **Manual of Clinical Oncology, 3rd Edition.** Boston, MA: Little Brown and Company, 1995.

Dow, Karen H. **Contemporary Issues in Breast Cancer.** Boston, MA: Jones and Bartlett, 1996.

Groenwald, S.L. **Cancer Nursing**. Boston, MA: Jones and Bartlett, 1992.

Groenwald, S.L. **Psychosocial Dimensions of Cancer**. Boston, MA.: Jones and Bartlett, 1992.

Haagensen, C.D. **Diseases of the Breast**. Philadelphia, PA: W.B. Saunders, 1986.

Harris, Jay R. **Diseases of the Breast**. Philadelphia, PA: J.B. Lippincott, 1996.

Holland, J., J. Rowland. **Handbook of Psycho Oncology**. New York, N. Y: Oxford University Press, 1998.

Glossary

It is important to understand the medical terminology related to your mate's diagnosis and treatments. The following is a list of the most common medical terms used in breast cancer. If you do not understand the technical language used by doctors or nurses, ask them to explain what they mean. Understanding the terms will enable you to be a more effective support partner.

A

Abscess - A collection of pus from infection.

Acini - The parts of the breast gland where fluid or milk is produced (singular: acinus).

Acute - Occurring suddenly or over a short period of time.

Adenocarcinoma - A form of cancer that involves cells from the lining of the walls of many different organs of the body. Breast cancer is a type of adenocarcinoma.

Adjuvant Treatment - Treatment that is added to increase the effectiveness of a primary treatment. In cancer, adjuvant treatment usually refers to chemotherapy, hormonal therapy or radiation therapy after surgery to increase the likelihood of killing all cancer cells.

Alkylating Agents - A type of chemotherapy drug used in cancer treatment.

Alopecia - Refers to hair loss as a result of chemotherapy or radiation therapy administered to the head. Hair loss from chemotherapy is temporary. Hair loss from radiation is usually permanent.

Amenorrhea - The absence or discontinuation of menstrual periods.

Analgesic - Medicine given to control pain; for example: Aspirin or Tylenol®.

Anesthesia - Medication that causes entire or partial loss of feeling or sensation.

Androgen - A male sex hormone. Androgens may be used in patients with breast cancer to treat recurrence of the disease.

Aneuploid - The characteristic of having either fewer or more than the normal number of chromosomes in a cell. This is an abnormal cell.

Anorexia - Severe, uncontrolled loss of appetite.

Antiemetic - A medicine that prevents or relieves nausea and vomiting, used during and sometimes after chemotherapy.

Antimetabolites - Anti-cancer drugs that interfere with the processes of DNA production, thus preventing cell division.

Areola - The circular field of dark colored skin surrounding the nipple.

Aspiration - Removing fluid or cells from tissue by inserting a needle into an area and drawing the fluid into the syringe.

Asymptomatic - Without obvious signs or symptoms of disease. Cancer may cause symptoms and warning signs; but, especially in its early stages, cancer may develop and grow without producing any symptoms.

Atypical Cells - Not usual; abnormal. Cancer is the result of atypical cell division.

Autologous - Coming from the same person.

Axilla - The armpit.

Axillary Dissection - Surgical removal of lymph nodes from the armpit. This tissue is then sent to the pathologist to determine if the breast cancer has spread outside of the breast. The number of nodes dissected varies during surgery. The physician can tell you how many nodes were removed.

Axillary Nodes - The lymph nodes in the axilla (underarm) that are cut out and examined during surgery to see if the cancer has spread past the breast. The number of nodes in this area varies.

B

Benign Tumor - An abnormal growth that is not cancer and does not spread to other parts of the body.

Bilateral - Pertains to both sides of the body. For example, bilateral breast cancer would be on both sides of the body, or in both breasts.

Biological Response Modifier - Treatment used which alters the body's natural response to stimulate bone marrow to make specific blood cells. Referred to as colony stimulating factors.

Biopsy - The surgical removal of a small piece of tissue or a small tumor for microscopic examination to determine if cancer cells are present. A biopsy is the most important procedure in diagnosing cancer.

Biotherapy - Treatments used to stimulate the body's immune system.

Blood Count - A test to measure the number of red blood cells (RBCs), white blood cells (WBCs) and platelets in a blood sample.

Bone Marrow - The soft, fatty substance filling the cavities of the bones. Blood cells are manufactured in the bone marrow. Chemotherapy will affect the bone marrow, resulting in a temporary decrease in the number of cells in the blood.

Bone Marrow Biopsy and Aspiration - A procedure in which a needle is inserted into the center of a bone, usually the hip, to remove a small amount of bone marrow for microscopic examination.

Bone Scan - The injection of a trace amount of radioactive substance into the bloodstream to illuminate the bones under a special camera to see if the cancer has spread to the bones.

Breast Cancer - If not removed from the body, a potentially fatal tumor because of its ability to leave the breast and go to other vital organs and continue to grow. These are breast cells that are abnormal with uncontrolled growth.

Breast Implants - A round or teardrop shaped sac inserted into the body to restore the shape of the breast. May be filled with saline water or synthetic material.

Breast Self-Exam (BSE) - A procedure to examine the breast thoroughly once a month to detect any changes or suspicious lumps. Exams should be practiced at the end of the period or seven days after the start of the period and be performed monthly at the same time.

ℭ

Calcifications - Small calcium deposits in breast tissue seen on mammography. The smallest object detected on mammography. Deposits are the result of cell death. Occurs with benign and malignant changes.

Cancer - A general term used to describe more than 100 different uncontrolled growths of abnormal cells in the body. Cancer cells have the ability to continue to grow, invade and destroy surrounding tissue, leave the original site and travel via lymph or blood systems to other parts of the body where they can set up new cancerous tumors.

Cancer Cell - A cell that divides and reproduces abnormally with uncontrolled growth. This cell can break away and travel to other parts of the body and set up another site, referred to as metastasis.

Clavicle - The collarbone.

Carcinoembryonic Antigen (CEA) - Blood test used to follow women with metastatic breast cancer to help determine if the treatment is working. This is not a test specific for cancer.

Carcinogen - Any substance that initiates or promotes the development of cancer. For example, asbestos is a proven carcinogen.

Carcinoma - A form of cancer that develops in tissues covering or lining organs of the body, such as the skin, the uterus, the lung or the breast.

Carcinoma In Situ - An early stage of development, when the cancer is still confined to the tissues of origin. It has not spread outside the area. In situ carcinomas are highly curable.

CAT Scan or CT Scan - An x-ray view of the body in sections.

Cell - The basic structural unit of all life. All living matter is composed of cells.

Cellulitis - Infection occurring in soft tissues. The surgical arm has an increased risk for cellulitis because of the removal of lymph nodes. Pain, swelling and warmth occur in the area.

Chemotherapy - Treatment of cancer by use of chemicals. Usually refers to drugs used to treat cancer.

Clinical Trial - Entering into a cancer treatment program that has proven to be effective after experiments. Evidence has proven potential effectiveness, and preliminary studies in humans suggest usefulness.

Combination Chemotherapy - Treatment consisting of the use of two or more chemicals to achieve maximum kill of tumor cells.

Combined Modality Therapy - Two or more types of treatments used to supplement each other. For instance, surgery, radiation, chemotherapy, hormonal or immunotherapy may be used alternatively or together for maximum effectiveness.

Complete Blood Count (CBC) - A laboratory test to determine the number of red blood cells, white blood cells, platelets, hemoglobin and other components of a blood sample.

Computerized Tomography Scans - Commonly called CT scans. These specialized x-ray studies indicate cancer or metastasis.

Cooper's Ligaments - Flexible bands of tissue that pass from the chest muscle between the lobes of the breasts which provide shape and support the breasts.

Core Biopsy - Removal (with a large needle) of a piece of a lump. The piece is sent to the lab to see if the lump is benign or malignant.

Cyst - An abnormal saclike structure that contains liquid or semi-solid material; is usually benign. Lumps in the breast are often found to be harmless cysts.

Cytology - Study of cells under a microscope that have been sloughed off, cut out or scraped off organs to microscopically examine for signs of cancer.

Cytotoxic - Drugs that can cause the death of cancer cells. Usually refers to drugs used in chemotherapy treatments.

𝔇

Detection - The discovery of an abnormality in an asymptomatic or symptomatic person.

Diagnosis - The process of identifying a disease by its characteristic signs, symptoms and laboratory findings. With cancer, the earlier the diagnosis is made, the better the chance for cure.

Differentiated - The similarity between a normal cell and the cancer cell; defines what degree of change has occurred. Cancer cells that are well differentiated are close to the original cell and are usually less aggressive. Poorly differentiated cells have changed more and are more aggressive.

Diaphanography (DPG) - A non-invasive procedure (no cutting) which uses ordinary light as an investigative tool to detect breast masses. Also called transillumination.

Diploid - The characteristic of having two sets of chromosomes in a cell. This is normal for a breast cell.

DNA - One of two nucleic acids (the other is RNA) found in the nucleus of all cells. DNA contains genetic information on cell growth, division and cell function.

Doubling Time - The time required for a cell to double in number. Breast cancer has been shown to double in size every 23 to 209 days. It would take one cell, doubling every 100 days, eight to ten years to reach one centimeter, 3/8 inch.

Ductal Carcinoma In Situ - A cancer, inside the ducts of a breast, that has not grown through the wall of the duct into the surrounding tissues. Sometimes referred to as a pre-cancer. Prognosis is good with in situ cancers.

Ductal Papillomas - Small noncancerous finger-like growths in the mammary ducts that may cause a bloody nipple discharge. Commonly found in women 45 to 50 years of age.

E

Edema - Excess fluid in the body or a body part described as swollen or puffy.

Endocrine Manipulation - Treating breast cancer by changing the hormonal balance of the body to prevent hormone-dependent cancer cells from multiplying.

Estrogen - A female hormone secreted by the ovaries which is essential for menstruation, reproduction and the development of secondary sex characteristics, such as breasts. Some patients with breast cancer are given drugs to suppress the production of estrogen in their bodies.

Estrogen Receptor Assay (ERA) - A test that is done on cancerous tissue to see if a breast cancer is hormone-dependent and may be treated with hormonal therapy. The test will reveal if your cancer is estrogen receptor positive or negative.

Excisional Biopsy - Surgical removal of a lump or suspicious tissue by cutting the skin and removing the tissue.

F

Familial Cancer - One occurring in families more frequently than would be expected by chance.

Fat Necrosis Tumor - Destruction of fat cells in the breast due to trauma or injury that can cause a hard noncancerous lump.

Fibroadenoma - A noncancerous, solid tumor most commonly found in younger women.

Fibrocystic Breast Changes or Condition - A noncancerous breast condition in which multiple cysts or lumpy areas develop in one or both breasts. It can be accompanied by discomfort or pain that fluctuates with the menstrual cycle. Large cysts can be treated by aspiration of the fluid they contain.

Fine Needle Aspiration - Procedure to remove cells or fluid from tissues using a needle with an empty syringe. Cells or breast fluid is extracted by pulling back on plunger and is then analyzed by a physician.

Flow Cytometry - A test done on cancerous tissues that shows the aggressiveness of the tumor. It shows how many cells are in the dividing stage at one time, commonly referred to as the 'S' phase, and the DNA content of the cancer, referred to as the ploidy. This reveals how rapidly the tumor is growing.

Frozen Section - A technique in which a part of the biopsy tissue is frozen immediately, and a thin slice is then mounted on a microscope slide, enabling a pathologist to analyze it in just a few minutes for a diagnosis.

Frozen Shoulder - Surgical shoulder which has severely restricted range of motion and is painful.

G

Galactocele - A clogged milk duct, often associated with childbirth.

Genes - Located in the nucleus of the cell, genes contain hereditary information that is transferred from cell to cell.

Genetic - Refers to the inherited pattern located in genes for certain characteristics.

H

Hematoma - A collection of blood that can form in a wound after surgery or an aspiration or from an injury.

Hormonal Therapy - Treatment of cancer by alteration of the hormonal balance. Some cancer will only grow in the presence of certain hormones.

Hormone - Secreted by various organs in the body, hormones help regulate growth, metabolism and reproduction. Some hormones are used as treatment following surgery for breast, ovarian and prostate cancers.

Hormone Receptor Assay - A diagnostic test to determine whether a breast cancer's growth is influenced by hormones or if it can be treated with hormones.

Hot Flashes - A sensation of heat and flushing that occurs suddenly. May be associated with menopause or some medications.

Hyperplasia - An abnormal, excessive growth of cells that is benign.

I

Intramuscular (I.M.) - To receive a medication by needle injection into the muscle of the body.

Immune System - Complex system by which the body protects itself from outside invaders which are harmful to the body.

Immunology - Study of the body's mechanisms of resistance against disease or invasion by foreign substances. The ability of the body to fight a disease.

Immunotherapy - A treatment that stimulates the body's own defense mechanisms to combat diseases such as cancer.

Immunosuppressed - Condition of having a lowered resistance to disease. May be a temporary result of lowered white blood cells from chemotherapy administration.

Incisional Biopsy - A surgical incision made through the skin to remove a portion of a suspected lump or tissue.

Inflammation - Reaction of tissue to various conditions which may result in pain, redness or warmth of tissues in the area.

Infiltrating Cancer - Cancer that has grown through the cell wall of the breast area, in which it originated, and into surrounding tissues.

Informed Consent - Process of explanation to the patient of all risks and complications of a procedure or treatment before it is done. Most informed consents are written and signed by the patient or a legal representative.

Intraductal - Residing within the duct of the breast. Intraductal disease may be benign or malignant.

Invasive Cancer - Cancer that has spread outside its site of origin and is growing into the surrounding tissues.

In Situ - In place, localized and confined to one area. A very early stage of cancer.

Infiltrating Ductal Cell Carcinoma - A cancer that begins in the mammary glands and has spread to areas outside the gland.

Intravenous (I.V.) - Entering the body through a vein.

Inverted Nipple - The turning inward of the nipple. Usually a congenital condition; but, if it occurs where it has not previously existed, it can be a sign of breast cancer.

L

Lactation - Process of being able to produce milk from the breasts.

Lesion - An area of tissue that is diseased.

Leukocyte - A white blood cell or corpuscle.

Leukopenia - A decrease in the number of white blood cells resulting in susceptibility to infection.

Linear Accelerator - A machine that produces high energy x-ray beams to destroy cancer cells.

Liver Scan - A way of visualizing the liver by injecting into the bloodstream a trace dose of a radioactive substance which helps visualize the organ during x-ray.

Lobular - Pertaining to the part of the breast that is furthest from the nipple, the lobes.

Localized Cancer - A cancer still confined to its site of origin.

Lump - Any kind of abnormal mass in the breast or elsewhere in the body.

Lumpectomy - A surgical procedure in which only the cancerous tumor and an area of surrounding tissue is removed. Usually the surgeon will remove some of the underarm lymph nodes at the same time. This procedure is also referred to as a tylectomy.

Lymphatic Vessels - Vessels that remove cellular waste from the body by filtering through lymph nodes and eventually emptying into the vascular (blood) system.

Lymph - A clear fluid circulating throughout the body in the lymphatic system that contains white blood cells and antibodies.

Lymph Gland - Also called a lymph node. These are rounded body tissues in the lymphatic system that vary in size from a pinhead to an olive and may appear in groups or one at a time. The principal ones are in the neck, underarm and groin. These glands produce lymphocytes and monocytes (white blood cells which fight foreign substances) and serve as filters to prevent bacteria from entering the bloodstream. They will filter out cancer cells but will also serve as a site for metastatic disease. The major ones serving the breast are in the armpit. Some are located above and below the collarbone and some in between the ribs near the breastbone. There are three levels of lymph nodes in the underarm area of the breast and another around the breast bone. Number of nodes vary from person to person. Lymph nodes are usually sampled during surgery to determine if the cancer has spread outside of the breast area.

Lymphedema - A swelling in the arm caused by excess fluid that collects after the lymph nodes have been removed by surgery or affected by radiation treatments.

M

Macrocyst - A cyst that is large enough to be felt with the fingers.

Magnification View - Special enlarged views used in mammography to magnify an area for greater detail of suspicious finding.

Magnetic Resonance Imaging (MRI) - A magnet scan; a form of x-ray using magnets instead of radiation. MRI gives a more clearly defined picture of fatty tissue than x-ray.

Malignant Tumor - A mass of cancer cells. These cells have uncontrolled growth and will invade surrounding tissues and spread to distant sites of the body setting up new cancer sites, a process called metastasis.

Mammary Duct Ectasia - A noncancerous breast disease most often found in women during menopause. The ducts in or beneath the nipple become clogged with cellular and fatty debris. The duct may have gray to greenish discharge, a lump that can be felt and can become inflamed, causing pain.

Mammary Glands - The breast glands that produce and carry milk by way of the mammary ducts to the nipples during pregnancy and breast feeding.

Mammogram - An x-ray of the breast that can detect tumors before they can be felt. A baseline mammogram is performed on healthy breasts usually at the age of 35 to establish a basis for later comparison.

Mammotest - Biopsy performed under mammography while breast is compressed and lesion is viewed by physician. Sample of lesion is removed using a large core needle and is then sent to lab to determine if it is benign or malignant.

Margins - The area of tissue surrounding a tumor when it is removed by surgery.

Mastalgia - Pain occurring in the breast.

Mastectomy - Surgical removal of the breast and some of the surrounding tissue.

>   **Modified Radical Mastectomy** - The most common type of mastectomy. Breast skin, nipple, areola and underarm lymph nodes are removed. The chest muscles are saved.

Prophylactic Mastectomy - A procedure sometimes recommended for patients at a very high risk for developing cancer in one or both sides.

Subcutaneous mastectomy - Performed before cancer is detected, removes the breast tissue but leaves the outer skin, areola and nipple intact. (This is not suitable with a diagnosis of cancer)

Radical Mastectomy (Halsted Radical) - The surgical removal of the breast, breast skin, nipple, areola, chest muscles and underarm lymph nodes.

Segmental Mastectomy (Partial Mastectomy/ Lumpectomy) - A surgical procedure in which only a portion of the breast is removed, including the cancer and the surrounding margin of healthy breast tissue.

Mastitis - Infection occurring in the breast. Pain, tenderness, swelling, redness and warmth may be observed. Usually related to infection and will respond to antibiotic treatment.

Menopause - The time in a woman's life when the menstrual cycle ends and the ovaries produce lower levels of hormones; usually occurs between the age of 45 and 55.

Metastasis - The spread of cancer from one part of the body to another through the lymphatic system or the bloodstream. The cells in the new cancer location are the same type as those in the original sites.

Microcalcifications - Particles observed on a mammogram that are found in the breast tissue appearing as small spots on the picture. Usually occur from calcium deposits caused by death of breast cells which may be benign or malignant. When clustered in one area, may need to be checked more closely for a malignant change in the breast.

Microcyst - A cyst that is too small to be felt but may be observed on mammography or ultrasound screening.

Micrometastasis - Undetectable spread of cancer outside of the breast that is not seen on routine screening tests. Metastasis is too limited to have created enough mass to be observed.

Multicentric - More than one origin or place of growth in the breast. These growths may or may not be related to each other.

Myleosuppression - A decrease in the ability of the bone marrow cells to produce blood cells, including red blood cells, white blood cells and platelets. This condition increases susceptibility to infection and produces fatigue.

N

Needle Biopsy - Removal of a sample of tissue from the breast using a wide-core needle with suction.

Necrosis - Death of a tissue.

Neoplasm - Any abnormal growth. Neoplasms may be benign or malignant, but the term is usually used to describe a cancer.

Nodularity - Increased density of breast tissue, most often due to hormonal changes in the breast, which causes the breast to feel lumpy in texture. This finding is called normal nodularity, and it usually occurs in both breasts.

Nodule - A small, solid mass.

𝕺

Oncogene - Certain stretches of cellular DNA. Genes that, when inappropriately activated, contribute to the malignant transformation of a cell.

Oncologist - A physician who specializes in cancer treatment.

Oncology - The science dealing with the physical, chemical and biological properties and features of cancer, including causes, the disease process and therapies.

One-Step Procedure - A procedure in which a surgical biopsy is performed under general anesthesia, and if cancer is found, a mastectomy or lumpectomy is done immediately as part of the same operation.

Oophorectomy - The surgical removal of the ovaries, sometimes performed as a part of hormone therapy.

Osteoporosis - Softening of bones that occurs with age, calcium loss and hormone depletion.

𝕻

Per Orally (P.O.) - To take a medication by mouth.

Palliative Treatment - Therapy that relieves symptoms, such as pain or pressure, but does not alter the development of the disease. Its primary purpose is to improve the quality of life.

Palpation - A procedure using the hands to examine organs such as the breast. A palpable mass is one you can feel with your hands.

Pathology - The study of disease through the microscopic examination of body tissues and organs. Any tumor suspected of being cancerous must be diagnosed by pathological examination.

Pathologist - A physician with special training in diagnosing diseases from samples of tissue.

Pectoralis Muscles - Muscular tissues attached to the front of the chest wall and extending to the upper arms. These are under the breast. They are divided into the pectoralis major and the pectoralis minor muscles.

Permanent Section - A technique in which a thin slice of biopsy tissue is mounted on a slide to be examined under a microscope by a pathologist in order to establish a diagnosis.

Platelet - A cell formed by the bone marrow and circulating in the blood that is necessary for blood clotting. Platelet transfusions are used in cancer patients to prevent or control bleeding when the number of platelets have decreased.

Ploidy - The number of chromosome sets in a cell.

Port, Life Port, Port-A-Cath - A device surgically implanted under the skin, usually on the chest, that enters a large blood vessel and is used to deliver medication, chemotherapy, blood products and also is used to obtain blood samples. A port is usually inserted if a person has veins in the arm which are difficult to use for treatment or if certain types of chemotherapy drugs are to be given.

Precancerous - Abnormal cellular changes that are potentially capable of becoming cancer. These early lesions are very amenable to treatment and cure. Also called pre-malignant.

Progesterone - Female hormone produced by the ovaries during a specific time in the menstrual cycle. Causes the uterus to prepare for pregnancy and the breasts to get ready to produce milk.

Progesterone Receptor Assay (PRA) - A test that is done on cancerous tissue to see if a breast cancer is hormone (progesterone) dependent and can be treated by hormonal therapy.

Prognosis - A prediction of the course of the disease–the future prospect for the patient. For example, most breast cancer patients who receive treatment early have a good prognosis.

Prolactin - Female hormone which stimulates the development of the breast and later is essential for starting and continuing milk production.

Prophylactic Mastectomy - Removal of high-risk breast tissue to prevent future development of cancer.

Prosthesis - An artificial form. In the case of breast cancer following mastectomy, a breast form that can be worn inside a bra.

Protocol - A schedule of selected drugs and treatment time intervals known to be effective against a certain cancer.

R

Radiation Therapy - Treatment with high energy x-rays to destroy cancer cells.

Radiation Oncologist - A physician specifically trained in the use of high energy x-rays to treat cancer.

Radiologist - A physician who specializes in diagnoses of diseases by the use of x-rays.

Radiotherapy - Treatment of cancer with high energy radiation. Radiation therapy may be used to reduce the size of a cancer before surgery or to destroy any remaining cancer cells after surgery.

Radiotherapy can be helpful in shrinking recurrent cancer to relieve symptoms such as pain and pressure.

Recurrence - Reappearance of cancer after a period of remission.

Regional Involvement - The spread of cancer from its original site to nearby surrounding areas. Regional cancers are confined to one location of the body. Regional involvement in breast cancer could include spread to the lymph nodes or to the chest wall.

Rehabilitation - Programs that help patients adjust and return to full productive lives. May involve physical therapy, the use of a prosthesis, counseling and emotional support.

Relapse - The reappearance of cancer after a disease-free period.

Remission - Complete or partial disappearance of the signs and symptoms of disease in response to treatment. The period during which a disease is under control. A remission, however, is not necessarily a cure.

Retraction - Process of skin pulling in toward breast tissue. Often referred to as dimpling.

Risk Factors - Anything that increases an individual's chance of getting a disease such as cancer. The risk factors for breast disease are a first degree relative with breast cancer, a high fat diet, early menstruation, late menopause, first child after 30 or no children.

Risk Reduction - Techniques used to reduce chances of getting a certain cancer. For example, reducing dietary fat may help prevent breast cancer.

$\mathcal{S}$

S Phase - Test that is performed to determine how many cells within the tumor are in a stage of division.

Sarcoma - A form of cancer that arises in the supportive tissues such as bone, cartilage, fat or muscle.

Secondary Tumor - A tumor that develops as a result of metastasis or spreads beyond the original cancer.

Secondary Site - A second site in which cancer is found. Example: cancer in the lymph nodes near the breast is a secondary site.

Side Effects - Usually describes situations that occur after treatments. For example, hair loss may be a side effect of chemotherapy, or fatigue may be a side effect of radiation therapy.

Staging - An evaluation of the extent of the disease, such as breast cancer. A classification based on stage at diagnosis which helps determine the appropriate treatment and prognosis. In breast cancer, it is determined by whether the lymph nodes are involved; if the cancer has spread to other parts of the body (through the lymphatic system or bloodstream) and set up distant metastasis; and the size of tumor. Five different stages are used in breast cancer with levels in each stage. Stage IV is the most serious.

Stellate - Appearing on mammography as a star-shape because of the irregular growth of cells into surrounding tissue. May be associated with a malignancy or some benign conditions.

Stereotactic Needle Biopsy - Biopsy done while breast is compressed under mammography. A series of pictures locate the lesion, and a radiologist enters information into a computer. The computer calculates information and positions a needle to remove the finding. A needle is inserted into the lump, and a piece of tissue is removed and sent to the lab for analysis. May be referred to as mammotest or core biopsy.

Stomatitis - Inflammation of the gastrointestinal tract creating discomfort and a potential for infection. May be caused by chemotherapy drugs.

Supraclavicular Nodes - The nodes located above the collarbone in the area of the neck.

ℭ

Thrombocytopenia - A decrease in the number of platelets in the blood resulting in the potential for increased bleeding and decreased ability for clotting.

Tissue - A collection of similar cells. There are four basic types of tissues in the body: epithelial, connective, muscle and nerve.

Transillumination - The inspection of an organ by passing a light through the tissues. Transmission of the light varies with different tissue densities.

Tumor - An abnormal tissue, swelling or mass, may be either benign or malignant.

Two-Step Procedure - When surgical biopsy and breast surgery are performed in two separate surgeries.

U

Ultrasound Examination - The use of high frequency sound waves to locate a tumor inside the body. Helps determine if a breast lump is solid tissue or filled with fluids.

Ultrasound Guided Biopsy - The use of ultrasound to guide a biopsy needle to obtain a sample of tissue for analysis by a pathologist.

Index

Supporting Someone
is the thermometer
of our love.

EduCare Library Series

Your Breast Cancer Treatment Handbook   **$21.95**
A woman's guide to the treatment of and recovery from breast cancer. Tear-out worksheets. (210 pages)

Helping Your Mate Face Breast Cancer   **$13.95**
A support partner's guide to helping a loved one face breast cancer. Tips for becoming an effective support partner. (133 pages)

Finding A Lump In Your Breast—
Where To Go . . . What To Do   **$14.95**
A guide for the woman who has a lump, suspicious mammogram, breast pain, breast discharge, high risk history or had breast cancer. Assessment worksheets, list of 410 medications and dietary products that cause breast changes, explanation of benign diseases and diagnostic tests with a glossary. (144 pages)

Solving The Mystery Of Breast Pain   **$ 9.95**
A guide for identifying causes of breast pain with assessment tools and steps for management.

Solving The Mystery Of Breast Discharge   **$ 9.95**
A guide for identifying causes of breast discharge. Assessment worksheets for identifying causes and steps for management.

Add Shipping $4.50 1 - 2 books
$1.00 each additional book

Discounts available to medical facilities for quantity orders.

To order, write or contact:
EduCare Publishing
P. O. Box 280305
Columbia, SC 29228
Voice: 803-796-6100 or Fax: 803-796-4150
E-Mail: educare@ix.netcom.com
Internet Site: www.cancerhelp.com/